PSYCHIATRY RECALL
2nd edition

RECALL SERIES EDITOR

LORNE H. BLACKBOURNE, M.D.
General Surgeon
Major, Medical Corps
United States Army
Fort Eustis, Virginia

PSYCHIATRY RECALL
2nd edition

BARBARA FADEM, PH.D.
Professor of Psychiatry
Department of Psychiatry
University of Medicine and Dentistry of New Jersey
Newark, NJ

STEVEN S. SIMRING, M.D., M.P.H.
Associate Professor of Psychiatry
Vice Chair for Education and Training
Department of Psychiatry
University of Medicine and Dentistry of New Jersey
Newark, NJ

LIPPINCOTT WILLIAMS & WILKINS
A **Wolters Kluwer** Company
Philadelphia • Baltimore • New York • London
Buenos Aires • Hong Kong • Sydney • Tokyo

Senior Acquisitions Editor: Neil Marquardt
Managing Editor: Beth Goldner
Marketing Manager: Scott Lavine
Production Editor: Caroline Define
Designer: Risa Clow
Compositor: Peirce Graphic Services
Printer: R.R. Donnelley & Sons

Printed in the United States of America

First Edition, 1997

Library of Congress Cataloging-in-Publication Data

Fadem, Barbara.
    Psychiatry recall / Barbara Fadem, Steven S. Simring.—2nd ed.
        p. ; cm.
    Includes index.
    ISBN 0-7817-4511-X
    1. Psychiatry—Examinations, questions, etc. I. Simring, Steven S. II. Title.
    [DNLM: 1. Mental Disorders—Examination Questions. 2. Psychiatry—Examination Questions. WM 18.2 F144p 2003]
    RC457.F33 2003
    616.89′0076—dc22

                                                                        2003060295

The publishers have made every effort to trace the copyright holders for borrowed material. If they have inadvertently overlooked any, they will be pleased to make the necessary arrangements at the first opportunity.

To purchase additional copies of this book, call our customer service department at **(800) 638–3030** or fax orders to **(301) 824–7390**. International customers should call **(301) 714–2324**.

Visit Lippincott Williams & Wilkins on the Internet: http://www.LWW.com. Lippincott Williams & Wilkins customer service representatives are available from 8:30 am to 6:00 pm, EST.

04 05 06 07 08
1 2 3 4 5 6 7 8 9 10

Contents

Preface

We wrote the second edition of *Psychiatry Recall* to give medical students the important information they will need during their third-year psychiatry clerkship and the USMLE Step 2 exam. This information is presented in a concise, manageable way. Like other books in the Recall series, the question and answer format will help students recall important information quickly. Our "typical patient" examples give students clinical "snapshots" of some of the most important syndromes. Because there is so little study time during clerkships, the recall questions in each chapter have been designed so that they can be completed during natural breaks in the day of a busy clerk.

In addition to sections on psychiatric syndromes, special sections pose questions concerning the role of psychological factors in medical illness and, alternatively, how medical illness affects psychological functioning. These sections will be useful to students in medical and surgical rotations as well as in psychiatry. Information contained in the sections on medicine and law and on medical ethics apply to current issues in all medical specialties.

Acknowledgments

We thank the staff of Lippincott Williams & Wilkins, especially Beth Goldner, for her helpful suggestions. We are deeply grateful to Dr. Charles Kellner, Chairman of the Department of Psychiatry of the New Jersey Medical School, for his support. Finally, we thank with great affection the dynamic, supportive, and involved New Jersey Medical School students: past, present, and future.

1 Introduction

USING THE STUDY GUIDE

Psychiatry Recall, 2nd edition, is designed to be used during the psychiatry clerkship. Although concise and useful, it is not a textbook. A standard psychiatry textbook should be used to clarify and increase your knowledge of a topic. *Psychiatry Recall* is organized in a self-study quiz manner. You can use it to evaluate how much information you know by covering the information in the right-hand column with the bookmark and answering the question in the left-hand column. The book is designed to provide short "bites" of information, so that when you have 5 free minutes on your psychiatry rotation, you can answer a page of questions.

STUDYING DURING THE PSYCHIATRY CLERKSHIP

Your learning objectives in the psychiatry clerkship are to
1. Understand the basic principles of psychiatry
2. Obtain information from patients
3. Make a diagnosis
4. Formulate a treatment plan

In addition, you need to be able to
1. Answer questions during patient rounds
2. Present a patient
3. Do a patient write-up
4. Pass the written examination

PRESENTING ON ROUNDS

Know everything about your patient, including
1. Psychiatric and medical histories
2. Physical examination results
3. Mental status
4. Patient complaints

STAYING OUT OF TROUBLE

1. If you do not know something, say so and pledge to find out the answer
2. Do not leave early

3. Do not argue with the staff
4. Volunteer to visit patients on your own time

ADMISSION ORDERS

On the patient's chart, admission orders (or transfer orders) appear in the "physician orders" portion. One preferred method of writing admission orders is the **seven "D's.**

Example:
    1. **Date** (e.g., 9/25/03)
    2. **Disposition** (e.g., admit to G Yellow, Dr. Simring)
    3. **Diagnosis (tentative) and condition,** e.g.,
        Acute schizophrenic episode
        Delusional, oriented × 2 (i.e., to person and place)
    4. **Directives**
        V/S (take vital signs): q 4 h (every 4 hours) or qd
          (every day)
        Activity: OOB (out of bed)
        Observation: Suicidal observation (one-on-one
          observation)
    5. **Diet** (e.g., diabetic)
    6. **Drugs** (meds; e.g., risperidone 1mg bid)
    7. **Diagnostics** (tests)
        Immediately (often in the emergency room), for
          example, chest x-ray (if not recorded within the last 6
          months), CBC with differential, SMA-7, blood
          alcohol and urine toxicology for drugs, urine test for
          pregnancy (women of childbearing age)
        The next morning (or within 24 hours), for example,
          serology for syphilis, thyroid function tests, Ca,
          Mg, P, EKG
        Special diagnostics, for example, medical consults,
          psychological tests, EEG

PROGRESS NOTES

Put everything in daily progress notes and sign the notes. If you forget to write something, you can add it later if you note this fact and date the later entry. One preferred method of writing progress notes is to **SOAP** the patient, as follows:

Example:
    10/28/03
    S: Subjective complaints (e.g., tired, wants to get out)
    O: Objective observations (e.g., cooperative, participating
      in all activities)

> **A: Assessment** (diagnosis and progress; e.g., thinking better organized, oriented × 3)
> **P: Plan** (e.g., haloperidol 5 mg/day, decrease medication, hold family meeting, contact outpatient facilities)

PSYCHIATRY PEARLS

What are the two most common behaviors that strongly suggest mania?	Excessive telephone calls and excessive spending (e.g., charge card bills)
What are the four "A's of schizophrenia?	Affect (blunted), ambivalence (simultaneous contradictory feelings), associations (loosened), autism (self-preoccupation)
What is the single best way to predict that an antipsychotic agent will cause parkinsonian symptoms?	If it is a low-dose, high-potency "typical" agent (like haloperidol)
What are the two most common signs of PCP (phencyclidine, "angel dust") use?	Vertical nystagmus and violent behavior
What two drugs are most closely associated with formication (feeling of bugs crawling on the skin)?	Cocaine use and alcohol withdrawal
What is the single most effective treatment for alcohol abuse?	Alcoholics Anonymous or similar self-help peer support program
How many "steps" are in most self-help peer support programs?	Twelve
Aside from depression, what are the two most common psychiatric causes of a positive dexamethasone suppression test?	Schizophrenia and dementia

Which medical illness is most likely to present with depression?

Pancreatic cancer

What group of drugs are indicated for obsessive-compulsive disorder?

Selective serotonin reuptake inhibitors (SSRIs) like fluvoxamine (Luvox) and fluoxetine (Prozac)

What is the single most effective way to differentiate between pseudodementia and dementia?

Give an antidepressant trial

What is a "grid" abdomen?

Evidence of multiple abdominal surgeries as seen in factitious disorder

What differentiates schizophrenia from schizoid and schizotypal personality disorders?

Psychosis in the first, but not in the second or third

What differentiates schizophrenia from schizophreniform disorder?

Presence of illness for more than 6 months in the former; 1 to 6 months in the latter

What are the three most common symptoms of borderline personality disorder?

Anger, feelings of boredom and emptiness, and the tendency to see others as all good or all bad (splitting)

What is the most common differential diagnosis of infantile autism?

Deafness

What two external factors are associated with midlife delusional disorder?

Deafness and immigrant status

What are the top five risk factors for suicide?

Serious prior attempt, older age, substance abuse or dependence, history of rage and violent behavior, male gender

What two psychoactive agents are most likely to cause agranulocytosis?

Carbamazepine (Tegretol) and clozapine (Clozaril)

What two methods can be used to induce symptoms of a panic attack in a panic disorder patient?

IV administration of sodium lactate and inhalation of carbon dioxide (have the patient breathe in and out of a paper bag)

What are the three most common reasons for involuntary commitment?

Suicidal, danger to others, life-endangering inability to care for self

What is the single best criterion to distinguish somatoform disorder from a hidden physical disorder?

Age—somatoform disorders usually begin at a young age, not late in life

What feature of the "Type A" personality is most closely associated with coronary artery disease?

Hostility

Which class of medically used drugs is most commonly associated with depression?

Antihypertensives

What are four medically used drugs that are commonly associated with anxiety?

L-dopa, insulin, anticholinergics, thyroid hormone

Where is the lesion most likely to be in a depressed patient with brain damage?

The left frontal lobe

What are the most commonly used antidepressants in the elderly?

Any of the SSRIs

SIG:E CAPS refers to which seven cardinal signs of major depressive disorder?

S: sleep (decreased)
I: interest (decreased)
G: guilt (increased)
E: energy (decreased)
C: concentration (decreased)
A: appetite (decreased)
P: psychomotor activity (decreased)
S: suicidal ideation (increased)

2

Classifying Psychiatric Disorders: The DSM-IV-TR

THE MULTIAXIAL SYSTEM

The *Diagnostic and Statistical Manual of Mental Disorders, 4th edition-Text Revision* (DSM-IV-TR) is published by the American Psychiatric Association and allows the diagnostic coding of specific psychiatric illnesses along a multi-axial system. To code a specific illness, the patient's clinical presentation and history are taken and matched with diagnostic criteria for that illness. The patient is then coded along five axes; a definitive diagnosis can be made using the first three axes.

What is Axis I?

Clinical disorders (e.g., schizophrenia, panic disorder, major depressive disorder)

Other disorders that may be a focus of clinical attention (e.g., medication-induced disorders, malingering)

What is Axis II?

Personality disorders: personal characteristics that may be overshadowed by the Axis I diagnosis but that are longstanding and enduring and often have a profound effect on patient functioning

Mental retardation: IQ 70 or below and other criteria

What is Axis III?

General medical conditions: physical illnesses that may be related to or affect the psychiatric problem

What is Axis IV?

Psychosocial and environmental stressors (e.g., death of a spouse, job loss, divorce)

What is Axis V?	**Global assessment of functioning (GAF):** quantification of how well the patient is functioning in everyday life using the GAF scale; for example, a GAF score of 91–100 indicates the patient is functioning in a superior fashion; a score of 1–10 indicates the patient is in serious danger of suicide or of hurting others

SUBTYPES AND SPECIFIERS-TR

What are subtypes?	Illnesses are broken down into subtypes depending on presentation of symptoms (e.g., schizophrenia, disorganized type).

What are specifiers?	1. Denote specific features of an illness (e.g., major depressive disorder with psychotic features)
	2. Define the severity of the illness (i.e., mild, moderate, or severe)
	3. Describe whether the illness is in partial remission or in full remission
	4. Disclose the patient's prior history of the particular psychiatric disorder
	5. Can be provisional if it is believed that full criteria for the disorder will be met over time
	6. Can include "not otherwise specified" (NOS) if the illness is atypical or does not fit clearly into the criteria for a specific disorder because
	   a. the disorder causes clear distress but is not listed in DSM-IV-TR,
	   b. it is not known whether an organic condition is responsible for the symptoms,
	   c. the disorder meets some of the criteria for one or more conditions, or
	   d. there is not enough information for full classification

DIAGNOSTIC GROUPINGS OF THE DSM-IV-TR

What are the disorders usually first diagnosed in infancy, childhood, or adolescence?

Mental retardation, learning disorders, motor skills disorders, communication disorders, pervasive developmental disorders, attention deficit and disruptive behavior disorders, feeding and eating disorders of infancy and early childhood, tic disorders, elimination disorders, other disorders of infancy, childhood, or adolescence

What disorders were formerly called "organic mental disorders"?

Delirium, dementia, and amnestic and other cognitive disorders

What disorders were formerly called "psychophysiologic disorders"?

Mental disorders due to a general medical condition

Substance-related disorders?

Alcohol-related disorders, amphetamine (or amphetamine-like)-related disorders, caffeine-related disorders, cannabis-related disorders, cocaine-related disorders, hallucinogen-related disorders, inhalant-related disorders, nicotine-related disorders, opioid-related disorders, phencyclidine (PCP)-related disorders, sedative-, hypnotic-, and anxiolytic-related disorders, polysubstance-related disorders, other or unknown substance-related disorders

Schizophrenia and other psychotic disorders?

Schizophrenia, schizophreniform disorder, schizoaffective disorder, delusional disorder, brief psychotic disorder, shared psychotic disorder ("folie à deux"), psychotic disorder due to general medical condition, psychotic disorder NOS

Mood disorders?

Major depressive disorder, dysthymic disorder, depressive disorder NOS, bipolar I disorder, bipolar II disorder, cyclothymic disorder, bipolar disorder NOS, mood disorder due to general medical condition, mood disorder NOS

Anxiety disorders?	Panic disorder (with or without agoraphobia), specific phobia, social phobia, obsessive-compulsive disorder (OCD), posttraumatic stress disorder (PTSD), acute stress disorder (ASD), generalized anxiety disorder, anxiety disorder due to a general medical condition, anxiety disorder NOS
Somatoform disorders?	Somatization disorder, conversion disorder, pain disorder, hypochondriasis, body dysmorphic disorder, undifferentiated somatoform disorder, somatoform disorder NOS
Factitious disorders?	Factitious disorder with predominantly psychological or physical signs and symptoms and with both psychological and physical signs and symptoms combined; factitious disorder NOS
Dissociative disorders?	Dissociative amnesia, dissociative fugue, dissociative identity disorder (multiple personality disorder), depersonalization disorder, dissociative disorder NOS
Sexual and gender identity disorders?	Sexual dysfunctions, paraphilias, gender identity disorders
Eating disorders?	Anorexia nervosa, bulimia nervosa, eating disorder NOS
Sleep disorders?	Primary sleep disorders (dyssomnias, parasomnias), sleep disorders related to another mental disorder, other sleep disorders
Impulse-control disorders not otherwise classified?	Intermittent explosive disorder, kleptomania, pyromania, pathological gambling, trichotillomania, impulse control disorder NOS
Adjustment disorders?	Adjustment disorder with depressed mood, with anxiety, with mixed anxiety and depressed mood, with disturbance of conduct, with mixed disturbance of emotions and conduct, unspecified

Personality disorders?

Paranoid, schizoid, schizotypal, antisocial, borderline, histrionic, narcissistic, avoidant, dependent, obsessive-compulsive, NOS

Other conditions that may be a focus of clinical attention?

Psychological factors affecting medical condition, medication-induced movement disorders, other medication-induced disorders, relational problems, problems related to abuse or neglect, additional conditions that may be a focus of clinical attention, (e.g., malingering)

PRACTICAL PSYCHIATRIC CLASSIFICATIONS

What is a psychotic disorder?

Psychosis is seen in many disorders, such as schizophrenia, and is characterized by loss of touch with reality, leading to problems in everyday functioning. Psychotic symptoms are exemplified by hallucinations and delusions, and are seen also in major mood disorders such as bipolar disorder and in the cognitive disorders, such as delirium.

What is a neurotic disorder?

Although the term "neurosis" is no longer used, it is a useful concept to describe a group of illnesses characterized by problems functioning in daily life and marked personal distress, but no break with reality. Neurotic symptoms (e.g., excessive worrying, obsessions, and compulsions) are seen in the somatoform and anxiety disorders as well as in the mood disorders.

What is an organic mental disorder?

This term has also fallen into disuse because of the theoretic difficulty in separating organic from nonorganic disorders, since all psychiatric symptoms are mediated by the brain. The term organic is still useful, however, to suggest gross anatomic abnormality or metabolic derangement. An organic cause of symptoms is likely if the patient
1. Is disoriented or confused
2. Has a sudden onset of symptoms
3. Has a significant medical illness
4. Has a history of abusing drugs

5. Has no family history or prior personal history of psychiatric illness

What is a personality disorder?

The personality disorders are conditions characterized by pervasive problems in social relationships. The patient usually feels no distress; it is her friends, coworkers, and relatives who complain. Although the patient may be upset over the consequences of such problems, she usually has no insight into the fact that her behavior is their cause.

3

Clinical Assessment: The Psychiatric Interview and Relevant Diagnostic Tests

EVALUATION

What information is obtained in the evaluation of a psychiatric patient?

1. The medical history
2. The psychiatric history
3. Current state of mental functioning using the mental status examination
4. Additional information using diagnostic tests such as psychological and neuropsychological tests, EEG, and other relevant assessment instruments

HISTORY

What information is obtained in the psychiatric history?

1. General information, including age, race, religion, occupation, education, and marital status; if patient cannot give her own information, identify informants and examine their possible biases
2. Chief complaint (i.e., What brings you here?)
3. Present illness
   Current symptoms
   Drug and alcohol use
   Current living situation in terms of other people, financial problems, and source of income
4. Past psychiatric and medical illness
   Previous treatment
   The relationship among events in the patient's past life (developmental psychiatric history, medical problems) and current emotional issues

What information is obtained in the developmental psychiatric history?

Questions about events in the patient's history are divided into family factors and developmental periods (i.e., prenatal, infancy, childhood, adolescence, and adult).

What is asked about the family?

Family structure
Family history of psychiatric illness, substance abuse, antisocial behavior
Parental level of education and occupation
Influence of religion
Siblings (birth order, health, occupations)

What is asked about the prenatal period and infancy?

Was the child wanted?
Were there difficulties in pregnancy and childbirth?
Were there problems with feeding, toilet training, sleeping?
Was the development of verbal and motor skills timely?

What is asked about childhood and adolescence?

Relationships with siblings?
Patient's personality in childhood?
What were peer relationships like in grade school?
What was the quality of human interactions, including sexual relationships, in adolescence?
History of emotional problems? Previous psychiatric contact?

What is asked about educational history?

Quality of academic performance?
Grades repeated or missed?
High school graduation or GED?
Post-high school education?

What is asked about occupational history?

Job changes?
Longest job held?
Military service?
Relationship with coworkers?
Does job match early ambitions?

How is this information obtained?

Using the clinical interview, the physician first establishes trust and confidence in the patient and then gathers medical, psychological, and social information to identify the patient's problem.

THE CLINICAL INTERVIEW

What are the techniques used to establish rapport with patients in the clinical interview?

Support, empathy, and validation, as well as the open-ended question

What is an open-ended question?

A question where the doctor exercises the least control. The one most likely to produce a good clinical relationship, aid in obtaining information about the patient, and not close off potential areas of pertinent information; for example, "Tell me about what happened last night"

What is the interview technique of support?

Expression of the physician's interest and concern for the patient; for example, "That must have seemed strange to you"

What is the interview technique of empathy?

Expression of the physician's personal understanding of the patient's problem; for example, "I understand that the hospital must seem scary to you"

What is the interview technique of validation?

Giving credence to the patient's feelings; for example "Many people would be frightened if they had the same experience you had"

What are the techniques used to obtain information in the clinical interview?

Facilitation, reflection, silence, confrontation, and recapitulation increase the probability of obtaining meaningful information

What is the interview technique of facilitation?

A basic technique to encourage the patient to elaborate on an answer; for example, "Tell me more"

What is the interview technique of reflection?

A variation of facilitation, in which the physician repeats the patient's response to encourage elaboration of the answer; for example, "You said that your heart began to beat rapidly as soon as you went outside?"

What is the interview technique of silence?

Waiting patiently for the patient to speak without interrupting him or her; the least controlling interviewing technique

What is the interview technique of confrontation?	Calling the patient's attention to inconsistencies in his or her responses or body language; for example, "You say that you are not nervous, yet you seem to me to be quite upset."
What is the interview technique of recapitulation?	Summing up the information obtained during the interview; for example, "Let's go over what happened last night. You felt very frightened and you called your sister. She came over and brought you into the hospital."

TRANSFERENCE IN THE PHYSICIAN-PATIENT RELATIONSHIP

What are transference reactions?	Unconscious emotional reactions of patients to their physicians, based in childhood parent-child relationships; they can interfere with the physician-patient relationship and with compliance with medical advice
What is positive transference?	The patient views the physician as good and has a high level of confidence in his or her abilities, even without the physician doing anything to earn it.
What is negative transference?	Unjustified resentment or anger of patients toward the physician if their desires and expectations are not realized; this may result in noncompliance with medical advice
What is countertransference?	Physicians' idiosyncratic reactions toward patients; physicians may feel guilty when they are unable to help a patient, or they may have particular feelings toward patients who remind them of a close relative or friend

PSYCHOLOGICAL TESTS

Why use psychological tests in evaluating psychiatric patients?	If you suspect that a patient may have a neuropsychiatric syndrome To measure a patient's intellectual functioning To help in diagnosing psychopathology To determine whether a patient is malingering

Which tests are used most commonly to assess neuropsychiatric functioning?

Bender Visual-Motor Gestalt Test is used to detect problems in perceptual-motor coordination by asking the patient to copy simple geometric drawings.

Halstead-Reitan Battery (HRB) is used to localize brain lesions.

Luria-Nebraska Neuropsychological Battery (LNNB) is used to identify brain dysfunction, such as dyslexia and to determine cerebral dominance.

Which test is used most commonly to assess intellectual functioning?

Wechsler Adult Intelligence Scale Revised (WAIS-R), by obtaining the patient's verbal, performance, and full-scale IQ scores

Which tests are used most commonly to assess personality characteristics and psychopathology?

Minnesota Multiphasic Personality Inventory (MMPI-2) is an objective "true-false" test particularly useful in detecting malingering ("faking good" or "faking bad"), and can be used by a clinician without special training.

Rorschach (inkblot) test is a projective test useful to identify the presence of thought disorders and the nature of defense mechanisms.

Thematic Apperception Test (TAT) asks the patient to make up stories based on drawings and is used to evaluate conflicts and emotions outside of the person's awareness.

Sentence Completion Test (SCT) is used to identify a patient's problems by the use of verbal associations (e.g., "I usually become frightened when I . . .").

OTHER TESTS USED IN THE EVALUATION OF PSYCHIATRIC PATIENTS

What is drug-assisted interviewing?

Sodium amobarbital (Amytal; 200–500 mg) or another sedative agent is administered IV at 15 to 50 mg/min until the patient is slightly sedated; in this state, acutely anxious, mute, psychotic, amnestic, or conversion disorder patients may be able to communicate with the therapist.

How are the EEG and Q (quantitative) EEG used diagnostically in psychiatry?	Differentiate organic from functional conditions (e.g., temporal lobe epilepsy from a psychiatric syndrome) by measuring (EEG) and quantifying (QEEG) electrical activity in the cortex Identify delirium—EEG slowing or increased fast activity Identify delirium tremens—increased fast activity Differentiate delirium from dementia (e.g., EEG is usually normal in Alzheimer and other irreversible dementias, abnormal in some reversible dementias)
How are EEG evoked potentials used in psychiatry?	To measure the electrical response of the brain to sensory stimuli and to evaluate vision, hearing, and other sensory function in infants, and brain responses in comatose patients and patients with demyelinating illness (e.g., multiple sclerosis)
How is neuroimaging used in psychiatry?	**Computed tomography** (CT) scan can identify structural abnormalities in the brain (e.g., generalized atrophy in Alzheimer disease, enlargement of lateral cerebral ventricles in patients with schizophrenia). **Magnetic resonance imaging** (MRI) helps to identify demyelinating disease; shows the biochemical condition of neural tissue as well as the anatomy without exposing the patient to ionizing radiation. **Positron emission tomography** (PET) scans, **functional MRI** (f-MRI), and **single photon emission computed tomography** (SPECT) can measure brain physiologic activity and identify areas of brain activity during specific tasks.

OTHER TESTS IN PSYCHIATRY

What is the dexamethasone suppression test (DST)?	Dexamethasone is a synthetic glucocorticoid that suppresses the secretion of cortisol in normal patients; in about half of patients with depression, this suppression is absent.

What is the DST used for in psychiatry?

Evidence indicates that patients with a positive DST (reduced suppression of cortisol after external administration of dexamethasone) respond well to treatment with antidepressant agents or to electroconvulsive therapy

Why is thyroid function measured in patients with mood disorders?

To screen for hypothyroidism, which can mimic depression, or hyperthyroidism, which can mimic anxiety; to screen for hypothyroidism associated with lithium treatment

Why are biogenicamine levels measured in patients with psychiatric symptoms?

Abnormalities in biogenic amines and their metabolites are found in some psychiatric syndromes:

Dopamine: body fluid levels of homovanillic acid (**HVA;** a dopamine metabolite) may be elevated in schizophrenics and decreased with antipsychotic drug treatment

Serotonin: body fluid levels of 5-hydroxyindoleacetic acid (**5-HIAA;** a serotonin metabolite) may be decreased in depressed or violent/impulsive people

Norepinephrine: body fluid levels of 3-methoxy-4-hydroxyphenyl-glycol (**MHPG;** a norepinephrine metabolite) may be decreased in depressed patients

What substances cause panic attacks in susceptible patients and are used to diagnose panic disorder?

IV administration of **sodium lactate;** inhalation of **carbon dioxide**

4

Clinical Assessment: The Mental Status Examination

What is the mental status examination?	A comprehensive survey of the current state of the patient's mental functioning
What is assessed on the mental status examination?	General presentation, state of consciousness, attentiveness, speech patterns, orientation, mood and affect, form of thought, thought content, perceptual ability, judgment, memory, intellectual functioning, and other mental variables

GENERAL PRESENTATION

What do you look for when evaluating the patient's appearance?	Posture: Is she standing up straight? Grooming: Is her hair combed? Appearance for age: Does she appear to be older than her chronological age? Clothing: Is she dressed appropriately?
How do you evaluate the patient's behavior?	Mannerisms: Does she show abnormal facial expressions? Psychomotor agitation or retardation: Does she seem physically "slowed down"? Tics: Does she show unusual, repetitive, nonproductive movements?
How do you evaluate the patient's attitude toward the examiner?	Reliable: Does she provide apparently correct historical information? Cooperative: Does she follow the examiner's instructions? Seductive: Is she behaving in a sexual fashion toward the examiner? Hostile: Does she seem angry at the examiner? Defensive: Does she seem to take the examiner's remarks personally?

SENSORIUM AND COGNITION

What do you look for when evaluating the patient's state of consciousness?	Level of alertness: Glasgow Coma Scale of 3 (coma) to 15 (completely alert) Lethargy or sleepiness: Does she seem mentally "slowed down"?
How do you determine if the patient is oriented to person, place, and time?	Person: ask her, What is your name? Who has come with you to my office? Whom do you live with? Place: ask her, Where are we now? Time: ask her, What is the year, season, time of day?
How do you evaluate her memory?	Immediate memory: ask her to remember three words and question her after 5 minutes Recent memory: ask her about her activities in the last 24 hours; verify information to rule out confabulation Remote memory: ask her about her place of birth, schools she attended, and historical information that most people would know
How do you determine if the patient can concentrate and pay attention?	See if she pays attention to you without being distracted by other stimuli. Ask her to repeat a string of three to six numbers forward and backward (digit span) and to spell the word "world" backward.
How do you evaluate the patient's cognitive ability?	See if she can read and write: ask her to read a simple paragraph of text Assess her spatial ability: ask her to copy a simple drawing of a triangle or a square See if her thinking is concrete: ask her to describe how a pear and an apple are alike See if she can think abstractly: ask her to explain the proverb "a rolling stone gathers no moss" Evaluate her intelligence, factual knowledge, and calculational ability: ask her how many years are in the term of a U.S. president, or how much is 9 times 7

What do you ask yourself to evaluate the patient's speech?	Is her speech too loud or too soft (i.e., how is its timbre)? Is her speech pressured (i.e., does she seem compelled to speak quickly)? Does she articulate clearly (i.e., is her speech readily understandable)? Does she have deficiencies in language (i.e., does she show poor use of words or poor vocabulary)?
What do you ask yourself to assess the patient's mood and affect?	Is she depressed (i.e., feel low, hopeless, helpless, suicidal)? Does she show mania (i.e., feel high, euphoric, irritable)? Does she show abnormalities in her external expression of mood (i.e., is her affect blunted, restricted, or flat)? Are her mood and affect similar (i.e., congruent)? Are her mood and affect appropriate to her current situation?

THOUGHT

What do you ask yourself to evaluate the patient's form or process of thought (associations between thoughts)?	Do her thought patterns make sense? Do her thoughts follow each other logically? Do her thoughts move rapidly from one to the other (i.e., flight of ideas)? Are her thoughts repeated over and over (i.e., perseveration)? Is she responding to the sounds rather than the meanings of words (i.e., echolalia)?
What do you ask yourself to evaluate the patient's thought content?	Does she have compulsive or obsessive thoughts (i.e., she says that she cannot get thoughts out of her head)? Does she have phobias (e.g., irrational fears)? Does she have hypochondriacal thoughts (e.g., the belief that she has cancer without physical evidence)? Does she have delusions (e.g., is convinced that the CIA is after her)? Does she have ideas of reference (e.g., the belief that someone on television is talking about her)?

Does she have thoughts of suicide or homicide?

What do you ask yourself to assess the patient's perception?

Does she have:
1. Illusions: misinterpretations of reality (e.g., thinking that a coat on a chair in a dark room is a man)
2. Hallucinations: false sensory perceptions (e.g., hearing voices, seeing nonexistent insects)

How do you assess the patient's judgment?

Give the patient hypothetical examples (e.g., What would you do if you found a stamped, addressed letter on the sidewalk?); assess the appropriateness of her response (e.g., "I would mail it.")

How do you assess the patient's insight?

Determine whether the patient understands that her symptoms are due to her illness.

How do you assess the patient's reliability?

Use the patient's responses, collateral information from friends or family members, and your clinical judgment to evaluate whether she is telling the truth or providing accurate information (e.g., about previous hospitalizations or drug use).

How do you assess the patient's level of impulse control?

Use the patient's history (e.g., arrests, fights) and current behavior to assess whether she is able to control her aggressive and sexual impulses.

5   Childhood Mental Disorders

PERVASIVE DEVELOPMENTAL DISORDERS

AUTISTIC DISORDER

Typical patient?	A 3-year-old boy pays little attention to adults, including his parents. Although he repeats certain words over and over in a stereotyped fashion, he does not speak voluntarily. He is fascinated with watching running water and must be restrained from constantly turning on the tap.
Characteristics?	Severe difficulties in communication but normal hearing; significant problems forming social relationships; repetitive behavior (e.g., spinning); self-destructive behavior (e.g., head banging) subnormal intelligence (IQ 70 and below) in about two thirds of patients; unusual abilities in some savant skills, such as exceptional calculation ability
DDx?	Congenital hearing impairment Schizophrenia with childhood onset Mixed receptive/expressive language disorder Psychosocial deprivation
Age of onset?	Before 3 years of age
Occurrence?	0.02% to 0.05% of children, although lesser forms are more common ("spectrum disorder"); three to five times more common in boys; when it occurs in girls, autistic disorder is more severe

Etiology?	Perinatal complications Cerebral dysfunction (e.g., seizures are often seen) Genetic component: the concordance rate for autism in monozygotic twins is at least 35% lower in dizygotic twins
Treatment?	Behavioral therapy to increase social and communicative skills, decrease behavioral problems, and improve self-care skills; provide support and counseling to the parents
Prognosis?	Most autistic children remain severely impaired in adulthood; few are able to work and live independently

ASPERGER DISORDER

Typical patient?	A 3-year-old boy can communicate verbally but shows few hand gestures, maintains poor eye contact, and has little interest in social interaction. Although he shows a variety of odd behavior patterns, his cognitive skills are age-appropriate.
Characteristics?	Significant problems forming social relationships, repetitive behavior, clumsiness in motor skills; in contrast to autistic disorder, little or no developmental language delay and relatively normal cognitive development
Age of onset?	First noticed at 3 to 5 years of age
Occurrence?	Incidence rate is unknown; more common in boys
DDx?	Autistic disorder Childhood schizophrenia Rett disorder (in girls) Obsessive-compulsive disorder Schizoid personality disorder
Etiology?	Unknown, but evidence of genetic etiology
Prognosis?	Better than for autistic disorder

RETT DISORDER

Typical patient?	After six months of normal development, an infant girl begins to lose her acquired skills. By 18 months of age, she shows little social interaction, an ataxic gait, and odd finger tapping and hand-wringing gestures.
Characteristics?	Diminished social interest and skills after a brief period of normal functioning, stereotyped odd body movements, psychomotor and mental retardation
DDx?	Autistic disorder Childhood disintegrative disorder Asperger disorder
Age of onset?	Before 4 years of age; usually between 5 and 48 months
Occurrence?	Almost always in girls; less common than autistic disorder
Prognosis?	Progressive and lifelong

CHILDHOOD DISINTEGRATIVE DISORDER

Typical patient?	A 3-year-old boy, whose previous functioning has been normal, stops speaking and interacting with others, can no longer dress himself, and begins to wet and soil himself.
Characteristics?	Regression in verbal, motor, and social development after at least 2 years of normal functioning; mental retardation
DDx?	Autistic disorder Rett disorder (in girls) Asperger disorder
Age of onset?	2 to 10 years of age
Occurrence?	Very rare, may be more common in boys
Prognosis?	Chronic and lifelong

ATTENTION DEFICIT AND DISRUPTIVE BEHAVIOR DISORDERS

ATTENTION DEFICIT HYPERACTIVITY DISORDER (ADHD)

Typical patient?
A 9-year-old boy gets into trouble at school because he constantly interrupts the teacher and disturbs the other students by talking and running around.

Characteristics?
Overactivity, self-control problems, limited attention span, prone to accidents, impulsiveness, emotional lability, irritability, normal intelligence

DDx?
Normal temperamental characteristics
Mood disorder
Anxiety disorder
Learning problems

Age of onset?
Before 7 years of age; lasts for at least 6 months

Typical history during infancy?
The child often showed:
1. Excessive crying
2. High sensitivity to stimuli
3. Sleep problems

Occurrence?
3% to 5% of children aged 5 to 12 years; up to five times more common in boys; must occur in at least two settings (e.g., in school and at home)

Etiology?
Genetic factors: higher concordance rate in siblings; parents have a higher incidence of antisocial personality disorder, somatization disorder, and alcoholism
Minor brain dysfunction, although there is no evidence of serious structural problems in the brain

Treatment?
CNS stimulants, which may lower activity level and increase attention span and the ability to concentrate:
1. **Methylphenidate** [Ritalin; Concerta (extended release); ≤ 60 mg/day in children older than 6 years]

2. **Dextroamphetamine sulfate** (Dexedrine: ≤ 40 mg/day in children older than age 3 years)
3. **Amphetamine/dextroamphetamine** [Adderall and Adderall XR (extended release): ≤ 3 mg/day in children older than 3 years]

Adverse effects of treatment?	Inhibition of growth and weight gain; both usually return to normal once the child stops taking the medication
Prognosis?	20% of children retain characteristics of ADHD, such as impulsiveness, into adulthood and remain at risk for mood and personality disorders; most children show complete remission during adolescence with few long-term negative effects; for "adult ADHD" continue treatment with CNS stimulants.

CONDUCT DISORDER

Typical patient?	A 9-year-old boy gets into trouble at school because he steals lunch money from other students and often starts fights, causing injury to the other students.
Characteristics?	Behavior which violates social norms, including aggressive behavior toward others and toward animals, lying and stealing, property destruction, serious deviation from societal and parental rules (e.g., truancy, running away)
DDx?	Mood disorder ADHD
Age of onset?	Before 10 years of age for childhood-onset type; after 10 years of age for adolescent-onset type
Occurrence?	6% to 16% of boys and 2% to 9% of girls younger than 18 years of age
Etiology?	History of abuse by caretakers Parental psychopathology and drug abuse CNS dysfunction; may be associated with ADHD

Treatment?	Structured environment, psychotherapy
Prognosis?	Associated with mood disorder, criminal behavior, and substance abuse in adulthood

OPPOSITIONAL DEFIANT DISORDER

Typical patient?	A 9-year-old boy gets into trouble at school because he refuses to do his classwork and often talks back to the teacher in a belligerent and hostile manner.

Characteristics?	A pattern of defiant, negative behavior toward adults; in contrast to conduct disorder, this behavior does not violate social norms; the child is:
	   Argumentative and angry
	   Easily annoyed and loses his temper
	   Resentful
	   Noncompliant with the requests of adults

DDx?	Normal oppositional behavior Conduct disorder Mood disorder
Age of onset?	Before 8 years of age
Occurrence?	2% to 16% of children of school age (up to age 18 years)
Etiology?	Defense against parental overprotection Parental psychopathology
Treatment?	Psychotherapy (individual, family, or behavioral)
Prognosis?	May progress to conduct disorder; remits in one quarter of children

TIC DISORDERS

TOURETTE DISORDER

Typical patient?	A 25-year-old man with a normal IQ and social relationships has experienced

shoulder twitching and lip smacking since 11 years of age. At 17 years of age, he began making intermittent braying noises and recently has begun to utter strings of curses in the middle of normal conversations with others.

Characteristics?

The display of involuntary movements and vocalizations: many motor tics [e.g., facial grimacing, eye blinking (often the first tic seen), yawning]; at least one vocal tic (e.g., barking or grunting); the involuntary use of profanity and obscene gestures may occur years after the initial motor tics are seen

Age of onset?

Before 18 years of age, usually between the ages of 7 and 8 years

Occurrence?

0.05% of children

Etiology?

Evidence of dysfunctional regulation of dopamine in the caudate nucleus
Genetic factors:
    Concordant in 50% of monozygotic twins and in 8% of dizygotic twins
    Three times more common in boys
    A genetic relationship with both ADHD and obsessive-compulsive disorder

Treatment?

1. Haloperidol (Haldol: 0.05–0.075 mg/kg/day) is the most effective treatment
2. Pimozide (Orap: < 10 mg/day) and atypical antipsychotics like risperidone (Risperdal) are also effective.
3. Clonidine (Catapres) can improve tics.

Prognosis?

Lifelong and chronic

CHRONIC MOTOR OR VOCAL TIC DISORDER

Characteristics?

The display of involuntary motor or vocal tics, but not both; all other characteristics are similar to those of Tourette disorder

ELIMINATION DISORDERS

ENURESIS

Characteristics?
Voiding of urine in inappropriate settings (e.g., in bed)

Age of onset?
Cannot be diagnosed before 5 years of age

Occurrence?
7% of boys, 3% of girls at 5 years of age

Etiology?
Often present in other family members
Physiologic factors (e.g., small bladder, naturally low nocturnal levels of antidiuretic hormone)
Psychological factors (e.g., psychological stress due to life-style changes such as moving or birth of a sibling)

Treatment?
1. For nighttime enuresis, the most effective treatment is behavioral (e.g., a buzzer and pad apparatus; the buzzer sounds when slight wetness is detected, waking the child)
2. Pharmacologic treatments may be used in the short term for intractable cases; these include imipramine (Tofranil) and antidiuretic compounds like intranasal desmopressin acetate (DDAVP)
3. Support and reassurance for the child and parents are useful in combination with other treatments

ENCOPRESIS

Characteristics?
Soiling (passage of feces) in inappropriate settings

Age of onset?
Cannot be diagnosed before 4 years of age

Occurrence?
1% of children at 5 years of age; three times more common in boys

Etiology?
Physiologic causes (e.g., lack of sphincter control, constipation with overflow incontinence)
Psychological causes (e.g., regression due to stress or power struggle with parents for autonomy)

Treatment?	1. For physiological causes: laxatives, stool softeners
	2. For psychological causes: psychotherapy, family therapy, and behavioral therapy

OTHER DISORDERS OF CHILDHOOD

SELECTIVE MUTISM

Typical patient?	A 9-year-old girl has not said a word at school for the past year, although she occasionally whispers to one friend. At home with her parents, she is appropriately talkative and social.
Characteristics?	A child who speaks in some social situations but not others; the child may communicate with hand gestures or other nonverbal means or may whisper; must be distinguished from normal shyness
Age of onset?	5 or 6 years
Occurrence?	Rare: up to 8 in 10,000 children May be more common in girls
Etiology?	Stressful life event is often present in the history
Treatment?	1. Family or behavioral therapy 2. Selective serotonin reuptake inhibitors (SSRIs) like fluoxetine (Prozac)
Prognosis?	Academic problems because of failure to speak in school 50% improve within 10 years; those who remain mute after 10 years of age have poorer prognosis

SEPARATION ANXIETY DISORDER

Typical patient?	Four months after moving to a new neighborhood, an 8-year-old girl refuses to go to the bathroom or go to sleep in her own bed alone. She also refuses to go to school. When questioned about her behavior, she seems anxious and tells you that she is scared that her mother will die.

Characteristics?	Overwhelming fear of the loss of parents, particularly the mother, which results in the child's refusal to be alone; parents are often overly concerned about the child
Age of onset?	Most commonly 7 to 8 years of age
Occurrence?	Up to 4% of grade-school children; less common in adolescents; no sex difference
Etiology?	History of a stressful life event (e.g., moving, death of a loved one) Genetic and/or learning factors Anxiety disorders are often present in the parents.
Treatment?	Family therapy is often effective. Gradual reintroduction to the school setting and individual psychotherapy Antidepressants, primarily imipramine (150-200 mg/day), have been useful.
Prognosis?	In adulthood, individual may be at risk for anxiety disorders, particularly agoraphobia.

REACTIVE ATTACHMENT DISORDER OF INFANCY OR EARLY CHILDHOOD

Typical patient?	A 20-month-old Romanian girl who has been in an orphanage since birth puts her arms out to every adult who comes into her room, even if she has never seen the person before.
Characteristics?	Disturbed social relatedness. Either nonresponsive to (inhibited type) or forms indiscriminate attachments to (disinhibited type) others. Shows developmental delays.
Age of onset?	Within the first few years of life
Occurrence?	Children exposed to repeated changes in environment and caregivers (e.g., in orphanages or foster homes)

Etiology?   Pathological care, including neglect or
                                 abuse

Treatment?   Improve the family situation with
                                 interventions, such as counseling;
                                 practical help with child care and
                                 educating caregivers in child-care skills

Prognosis?   Some recover completely. Others remain
                                 impaired in social interactions. The
                                 disinhibited type has a better prognosis
                                 than the inhibited type.

6 Cognitive Disorders

DELIRIUM

CHARACTERISTICS

Typical patient?
One week after an acute myocardial infarction, a 56-year-old man with no prior history of psychiatric illness becomes agitated and complains of seeing strange animals in his room.

What is it?
Clouding of consciousness and difficulty with orientation due to central nervous system dysfunction

What aspects of orientation are most affected?
Time and place; orientation to person is the last to be affected

How does the patient appear?
Hyperactive or hypoactive, anxious, and confused

Other characteristics?
Illusions and hallucinations (often visual), diurnal variation in symptoms (often worse at night), sleep disturbances, and autonomic dysfunction

DDX

What other conditions mimic delirium?
Dementia, psychosis, and depression

OCCURRENCE

How common is it?
It is the most common psychiatric syndrome seen in hospitalized patients.

In which hospitalized patients is it most commonly seen?
It occurs more commonly in surgical and coronary intensive care units.

What age groups are at highest risk?	The elderly and children

ETIOLOGY

What are the four most common causes of delirium?	1. **Diseases of the central nervous system** (e.g., meningitis, encephalitis) 2. **Systemic illnesses** (e.g., liver, kidney, cardiovascular, or lung disease) 3. **Drug abuse** (e.g., phencyclidine, sedatives, alcohol) 4. **Withdrawal** of sedative drugs (e.g., alcohol, benzodiazepines, barbiturates)
Other causes?	Fever, sensory deprivation, postoperative conditions, and anticholinergic medications
Treatment?	Remove the cause and delirium will remit.
Prognosis?	1. Good if the cause can be removed 2. Can progress to dementia or death if untreated

OVERVIEW OF THE DEMENTIAS

CHARACTERISTICS

What are they?	Conditions characterized by gradual loss of memory and intellectual abilities
Are movement disorders present?	Movement disorders are seen in subcortical dementias (Huntington disease, Parkinson disease, human immunodeficiency virus [HIV] encephalopathy).
What psychopathology is commonly seen?	Anxiety and depression in the early stages

ETIOLOGY

What is the most common cause of dementia?	Alzheimer disease (at least 50% of all dementias)

Other common causes?	Multiple small infarctions in the brain (vascular dementia) Lewy body disease Primary or metastatic tumor Huntington disease Parkinson disease
How does HIV infection cause dementia?	It can infect the brain directly, causing cortical atrophy, inflammation, and demyelination; or dementia can result from cerebral lymphoma or opportunistic brain infections
What is the prognosis for patients with HIV dementia?	Death occurs in most patients within 6 months
What other conditions cause dementia?	Head trauma, multiple sclerosis, Creuzfeldt-Jakob disease, Pick disease
What is the age group in which dementia most commonly occurs?	The elderly

PROGNOSIS

What percentage of dementias are reversible?	About 15% of cases
What is the prognosis for the rest?	Memory loss and confusion (with or without psychosis) progresses to coma and death

DEMENTIA OF THE ALZHEIMER TYPE (ALZHEIMER DISEASE)

CHARACTERISTICS

Typical patient?	A 72-year-old retired schoolteacher is alert but does not know what month it is, nor can she precisely identify the man next to her (her husband).
Most common characteristics?	Normal consciousness Memory loss Language difficulties
What other problems occur?	Changes in personality (e.g., anger, paranoia) and mood (e.g., depression)

DDX

How do you know the deficits are not caused by normal aging?	**Normal aging** is associated with reduction in the ability to learn new things quickly and a general slowing of mental processes; in contrast to Alzheimer disease, changes with normal aging do not interfere with normal life
With what two conditions is Alzheimer disease most commonly confused?	1. **Depression** ("pseudodementia") is associated often with cognitive disturbances (e.g., confusion, memory problems) in the elderly 2. **Delirium** caused by illness or medications
Occurrence?	At least 20% of people older than 80 years of age have significant dementia

ETIOLOGY

Gross neuroanatomic findings?	Enlarged ventricles, diffuse atrophy, flattened sulci
Microscopic neuroanatomic findings?	Senile (amyloid) plaques and neurofibrillary tangles (seen also in Down syndrome and to a lesser extent in normal aging), loss of cholinergic neurons in the basal forebrain, neuronal loss and degeneration in the hippocampus and cortex
Neurophysiologic abnormalities?	Reduction in brain levels of choline acetyltransferase (needed to synthesize acetylcholine), abnormal processing of amyloid precursor protein, decreased membrane fluidity due to abnormal regulation of membrane phospholipid metabolism
What neurotransmitter abnormalities are there?	Hypoactivity of acetylcholine and norepinephrine, abnormal activity of somatostatin, vasoactive intestinal peptide, and corticotropin
What genetic factors have been implicated?	Having a close relative with Alzheimer disease, abnormalities of chromosomes 1, 14, or 21, possession of at least one copy of the E_4 gene on chromosome 19

TREATMENT

Psychosocial treatment?
Structured environment, nutritious diet, exercise, and recreational therapy for the patient; psychotherapy and support groups for family caretakers

Pharmacologic treatment?
Antianxiety, antidepressant, and antipsychotic agents to relieve associated symptoms
Acetylcholinesterase inhibitors like:
Tacrine (Cognex, 40 to 160 mg/day)
Donepezil (Aricept, 5 to 10 mg/day)
Rivastigmine (Exelon, 6 to 12 mg/day)
Galantamine (Reminyl, 16 to 32 mg/day)

PROGNOSIS

How does the illness progress?
Slow onset, steady and progressive deterioration of cognitive function, coma, and death

What is the progression of functional loss?
Memory is affected first (recent worse than remote), followed second and third by language (e.g., difficulty finding the right word) and spatial ability (e.g., difficulty copying a simple drawing), respectively

Life expectancy?
Approximately 8 years after diagnosis

VASCULAR DEMENTIAS

Typical patient?
An 80-year-old man whose mental functioning has been normal suddenly cannot remember how to turn on the television or what the phone is used for.

How does the presentation differ from Alzheimer disease?
1. Sudden rather than gradual onset of cognitive dysfunction
2. Stepwise rather than steady deterioration of function
3. Better preservation of the patient's personality characteristics
4. May have focal neurologic symptoms

DDx?	Delirium
What percentage of dementias are vascular in origin?	15% to 30% of dementias
Is there a gender difference?	Men are at higher risk than women
Etiology?	Multiple, small cerebral infarctions as a result of atherosclerosis, hypertension, valvular heart disease, or arrhythmias
Treatment?	Reduce risk factors associated with cerebrovascular disease (i.e., hypertension, excessive body weight, smoking, alcohol abuse, arrhythmias).
Prognosis	There is an abrupt loss of function with each cerebral infarction.

AMNESTIC DISORDERS

Typical patient?	An alert 50-year-old man with a history of alcoholism tells you that he graduated from high school in 1999.

CHARACTERISTICS

What are they?	Disorders characterized by memory loss with little or no other cognitive impairment
What types of memory loss are seen?	Both **retrograde** (i.e., memory for past events, particularly the recent past) and **anterograde** amnesia (i.e., inability to put down new memories) occur; the patient often fabricates forgotten information to cover up memory loss (i.e., confabulation)
Level of consciousness?	Normal
DDx?	Dementia, delirium, normal aging, dissociative disorders, and factitious disorder (see Chapter 12)

ETIOLOGY

What is the primary cause of amnestic disorder?

Thiamine deficiency resulting in destruction of mediotemporal lobe structures (e.g., mammillary bodies and hippocampus) as a result of long-term alcohol abuse; Wernicke's encephalopathy (acute delirium) followed by Korsakoff syndrome (chronic amnestic disorder)

What other conditions are most likely to cause amnestic disorder?

1. Head injury, cerebrovascular disease, or infection involving the temporal lobes (e.g., herpes simplex encephalitis)
2. Exposure to neurotoxins

Treatment and prognosis?

Based on the underlying cause

Substance-Related Disorders

OVERVIEW

What is the definition of:

Substance abuse?	A pattern of abnormal drug use leading to impairment of social, physical, or occupational functioning and often characterized by tolerance or dependence
Tolerance?	The need for increased amounts of the substance to gain the same positive effects
Cross-tolerance?	When tolerance develops to one substance as the result of use of another substance
Substance dependence?	Substance abuse plus tolerance and withdrawal symptoms when the drug is discontinued
What are the most commonly used and abused substances (% current users/% ever used)?	Caffeine: 75%/80% Alcohol: 50%/85% (13% abusers) Nicotine: 30%/55% Marijuana: 10%/33% Cocaine: 3%/12% Amphetamines: 1.3%/7% Heroin: 0.2%/1.3%
What are the most common psychiatric syndromes associated with substance abuse?	Mood disorders, anxiety disorders, borderline and antisocial personality disorders, schizophrenia, conduct disorder in adolescents

CAFFEINE

Type of drug	Stimulant
Major neurotransmitter system involved?	Dopamine

Found in?   Coffee (125 mg/cup), tea (65 mg/cup),
                                       cola (40 mg/cup), nonprescription
                                       stimulants, and diet agents

Physical effects?   Alertness, central nervous system and
                                       cardiac stimulation, and increased
                                       urination, peristalsis, and secretion of
                                       gastric acid

Adverse effects?   Agitation, insomnia, cardiac arrhythmias,
                                       increased blood pressure

Withdrawal symptoms?   Headache, slight weight gain, lethargy,
                                       depression

**Treatment of withdrawal   Analgesics to control headache
symptoms?**

**Initiation and maintenance   Substitute decaffeinated coffee or tea
of abstinence?**

NICOTINE

Type of drug?   Stimulant

**Major neurotransmitter   Dopamine
system involved?**

Laboratory findings?   Increased levels of cotinine (nicotine
                                       metabolite) in body fluids (used by
                                       insurance companies to identify smokers)

High-risk groups?   Increased use in teenagers, women, and
                                           African-Americans overall (but
                                           decreased use in African-American
                                           teenagers)
                                       Psychiatric patients smoke at a higher
                                           rate than the general population.

Physical effects?   Increased peristalsis; vasoconstriction of
                                       peripheral blood vessels

**Adverse effects of   Cancer of lung, pharynx, bladder; cardiac
smoking?**   and circulatory diseases; tremor; low birth
                                       weight in infants of mothers who smoke;
                                       decreases life expectancy more than any
                                       other substance, including alcohol

Withdrawal symptoms?	Headache, lethargy, depression, weight gain
Treatment of withdrawal symptoms?	Analgesics to control headache, nicotine-containing gum, patch, or nasal spray
Initiation and maintenance of abstinence?	Peer support groups (80% relapse rate within 2 years overall; 66% relapse rate among members of peer support groups) Support from a spouse, child, or non-smoking physician

ALCOHOL

Type of drug?	Sedative
Major neurotransmitter involved?	GABA (γ-aminobutyric acid)
Laboratory findings?	Elevated blood alcohol levels (see later); elevated (> 30 units) γ-glutamyltransferase (GGT)
High-risk groups?	The 21- to 34-year-old age-group African-Americans, Native Americans, Eskimos, Protestants (except fundamentalists), and Catholics
Use in women versus men?	Less alcohol use in women than in men Use is increasing among women More serious health effects in women Onset at a later age in women Women may be more secretive about their drinking habits
What conditions are frequently seen in the developmental history of the patient?	Attention deficit hyperactivity disorder, conduct disorder
Physical effects?	Sedation, elevated mood
Adverse social effects?	Half of all traffic fatalities and homicides and one quarter of all suicides are correlated with alcohol use; family, work, and legal problems

Adverse physiologic effects?	Liver dysfunction (e.g., cirrhosis) Gastrointestinal symptoms (e.g., ulcers) Thiamine deficiency resulting in Wernicke and Korsakoff syndromes (see Chapter 6) Reduced life expectancy Fetal alcohol syndrome (including facial abnormalities, reduced height and weight, and mental retardation) in infants of alcohol-using mothers
Treatment of physiologic adverse effects?	Thiamine 100 mg IM initially and 200 mg/day for 4 days; restore nutritional state
What is intoxication?	Legal definition: 0.08%–0.15% blood alcohol concentration (BAC), depending on individual state laws Coma occurs at a BAC of 0.40%–0.50% in nonalcoholics Tolerance is likely if symptoms of intoxication are not seen with BAC of 0.10%
Withdrawal symptoms?	Tremor, tachycardia, hypertension, malaise, nausea, seizures, delirium tremens ("DTs"; see Chapter 6)
Treatment of withdrawal symptoms?	Benzodiazepines or barbiturates: For anxiety, chlordiazepoxide (25–100 mg) or diazepam (10–20 mg) every 4 hours; for delirium, dose every hour For seizures, 100–150 mg phenobarbital IM or 5–10 mg diazepam IV
What is the most effective treatment for initiation and maintenance of abstinence?	Voluntary peer support 12-step programs such as Alcoholics Anonymous
Other methods for initiation and maintenance of abstinence?	Disulfiram (Antabuse; 125–500 mg/day) causes acetaldehyde accumulation in the blood, resulting in intense nausea, headache, and flushing when the patient subsequently drinks alcohol; is most useful in highly motivated patients Individual or group psychotherapy and family therapy may be useful, particularly if the spouse participates.

OPIATES

Type of drug?	Sedatives and analgesics; group includes morphine, heroin, methadone, codeine
Major neurotransmitter systems involved?	Opioid receptors, dopamine
Laboratory findings?	1. Most opiates present in urine and blood for 12–36 hours after use 2. Methadone can be detected for 2–3 days after use 3. Fentanyl is not identified by usual tests for opiates
High-risk groups?	Chronic pain patients Residents of urban ghettos
Physical effects?	Analgesia, euphoria, sedation, constricted pupils (miosis)
Adverse effects?	Respiratory depression leading to coma and death
Treatment of adverse effects?	For overdose, short-acting opioid antagonist, naloxone (Narcan) 0.4 mg IV; five doses at 3-minute intervals, more if needed
Withdrawal symptoms?	Anxiety, insomnia, anorexia, sweating, fever, rhinorrhea, piloerection, gastrointestinal problems
Is withdrawal from opioids life threatening?	Death from withdrawal is rare unless a serious physical illness is present
Treatment of withdrawal symptoms?	Methadone detoxification (10 mg PO q.i.d. for 7 days; reduce to 10%–20% of this dose when patient is stable) Clonidine (0.15 mg b.i.d.) suppresses autonomic withdrawal symptoms
What is used for the initiation and maintenance of abstinence?	Methadone, a synthetic opiate, can be substituted for heroin for detoxification or maintenance because it suppresses heroin withdrawal symptoms

How does methadone compare with heroin with respect to dependence and tolerance?	Methadone use also results in dependence and tolerance
How does methadone compare with heroin with respect to duration of action, mode of administration, and effects?	Methadone has a longer duration of action, is taken orally rather than injected, is less sedating, and has less euphoric action. These features allow the person using methadone to lead a relatively normal life
Other methods for the initiation and maintenance of abstinence?	Naltrexone (Revia) to block the potential effects of opiates; voluntary peer support 12-step programs, such as Narcotics Anonymous

BARBITUATES AND BENZODIAZEPINES

Type of drug?	Sedative
Major neurotransmitter system involved?	GABA
Laboratory findings?	Specific sedatives or their metabolites can be identified in blood; urine tests are positive for up to 1 week
High-risk groups?	People with insomnia or anxiety disorders Users of other drugs: To boost the effects of opiates To modify the anxiety-provoking effects of phencyclidine (PCP), LSD, and amphetamines
Physical effects?	Sedation, anesthesia, antianxiety, anticonvulsant
Adverse effects?	Depression of the respiratory system (less with benzodiazepines), high addiction potential, alcohol interactions
Treatment of adverse effects?	Gradual reduction in dosage of the abused drug
Withdrawal symptoms?	Anxiety, seizures, delirium, life-threatening cardiovascular collapse (withdrawal from barbiturates)

Treatment of withdrawal symptoms?	Hospitalization; substitution of long-acting barbiturates (such as phenobarbital) or benzodiazepines (diazepam) for the more commonly abused short-acting types
Initiation and maintenance of abstinence?	Psychological support, behavior therapy

AMPHETAMINES

Type of drug?	Stimulants, including dextroamphetamine (Dexedrine), methamphetamine (Desoxyn), and methylphenidate (Ritalin); "ice" is a street form of methamphetamine
Indications?	Attention deficit hyperactivity disorder in children and narcolepsy; also used for refractory depression and the short-term treatment of obesity if state laws permit
Major neurotransmitter system involved?	Dopamine
Laboratory findings?	Present in urine for 1–2 days
High-risk groups?	Professionals Occupations requiring late-night work (e.g., musicians, students) 18- to 25-year-olds
Physical effects?	Stimulants act rapidly, have euphoric action, reduce fatigue, increase performance, elevate pain threshold, reduce appetite, dilate pupils, and increase libido
Adverse effects?	Tachycardia, cardiomyopathy (rare), hypertension, fever, psychotic symptoms that may resemble those of schizophrenia
Treatment of adverse effects?	Benzodiazepines (e.g., diazepam 10–20 mg PO) to treat agitation Antipsychotic to treat psychotic symptoms (e.g., haloperidol 5–10 mg IM or 10 mg PO)

Withdrawal symptoms?	Post-use "crash," including depression, fatigue, headache, hunger, constricted pupils, and psychological craving
Treatment of withdrawal symptoms?	Medical and psychological support
Initiation and maintenance of abstinence?	No specific treatment has proven effective

COCAINE

Type of drug?	Stimulant
Major neurotransmitter system involved?	Dopamine
Laboratory findings?	Increased levels of benzoylecgonine (a cocaine metabolite) for 1–3 days in occasional users, 7–12 days for heavy users
High-risk groups?	Urban professionals, in expensive, pure form (snorted) Residents of urban ghettos, in inexpensive crack form (smoked) Cocaine use has declined since its peak in 1985
Physical and psychological effects?	Dilated pupils. Intense euphoria that lasts up to 1 hour
Adverse effects?	**Physical:** cardiac arrhythmias, hypertension, nasal problems, seizures **Psychological:** aggressiveness, agitation, hypersexuality, irritability, impaired judgment, psychotic symptoms [e.g., tactile hallucinations ("cocaine bugs")] Hyperactivity and growth retardation are seen in newborns with use during pregnancy
Treatment of adverse effects?	Medical support to treat cardiac symptoms and seizures, which may result in anoxia Benzodiazepines to treat agitation (e.g., diazepam 10–20 mg PO) Antipsychotics to treat psychotic symptoms (e.g., haloperidol 5–10 mg IM or 10 mg PO)

Withdrawal symptoms?	Post-use "crash," including fatigue, headache, depression, malaise, constricted pupils, and severe psychological craving
Treatment of psychological withdrawal symptoms (craving)?	Desipramine (Norpramin 200–250 mg/day)
Initiation and maintenance of abstinence?	Not established

CANNABIS (TETRAHYDROCANNABINOL): MARIJUANA

Type of drug?	Hallucinogen
Major neurotransmitter system involved?	Serotonin (5-HT)
Laboratory findings?	Cannabinoid metabolites in urine for 7–10 days; up to 28 days in heavy users
High-risk groups?	Currently use is increasing in teenagers; decreased use through 1980s
Can marijuana legally be prescribed by a physician?	No, but at least two states permit limited medical use to treat glaucoma and cancer-related nausea and vomiting.
Physical effects?	Orthostatic hypotension and tachycardia
Psychological effects?	Euphoria, relaxation
Adverse effects?	**Low doses:** impairs memory and complex motor activity, alters sensory and time perception, causes conjunctival reddening, and may increase appetite and sexual desire **High doses:** psychotic symptoms, paranoia **Chronic use:** decreased sexual functioning, lung problems associated with smoking, and a decrease in motivation (the "amotivational syndrome")
Treatment of adverse effects?	Calm the patient by "talking him down"; benzodiazepines (diazepam, 10–15 mg)

Withdrawal symptoms and treatment?	None
Initiation and maintenance of abstinence?	Education

LYSERGIC ACID DIETHYLAMIDE (LSD)

Type of drug?	Hallucinogen
Major neurotransmitter involved?	5-HT
Laboratory tests?	Urine toxicology results are positive for LSD
Physical effects?	Last between 8 to 12 hours; include profuse perspiration, blurred vision, pupil dilation, tachycardia, tremor, and palpitations
Psychological effects?	Altered perception and emotions
Adverse effects?	"Bad trips" (i.e., panic reactions that may include psychotic symptoms); flashbacks (i.e., a reexperience of the associated sensations in the absence of the drug); psychiatric problems; long-term cognitive impairment may occur
Treatment of adverse effects?	Calm the patient by "talking him down"; hospitalization and medical maintenance; benzodiazepines (diazepam, 10–20 mg orally) to decrease agitation; antipsychotics (e.g., haloperidol 5–10 IM or 10 PO) to treat psychotic symptoms
Withdrawal symptoms and treatment?	None
Initiation and maintenance of abstinence?	Education

PHENCYCLIDINE PIPERIDINE (PCP), "ANGEL DUST"

Type of drug?	Hallucinogen-like dissociative anesthetic

Major neurotransmitters involved?	Glutamate, dopamine
Laboratory findings?	PCP may be found in urine for more than 1 week; elevated serum glutamic-oxaloacetic acid; elevated creatinine phosphokinase
Route of administration?	Smoked with marijuana or tobacco cigarette
Physical effects?	Long-lasting effects: detectable in blood for > 1 week; hypertension, hyperthermia, and nystagmus (abnormal eye movements); consumption of more than 20 mg may cause convulsions, coma, and death
Psychological effects?	Fantasies, euphoria, episodes of extremely violent behavior
Adverse effects?	**Short-term effects:** PCP psychosis, including auditory and visual hallucinations, distortions of body image, time and space, aggressiveness **Long-term effects:** memory loss, lethargy, reduced attention span
Treatment of adverse effects?	Same as for LSD
Withdrawal symptoms and treatment?	None
Initiation and maintenance of abstinence?	Education

8 Schizophrenia

CHARACTERISTICS

Typical patient?

A 35-year-old woman tells you that her neighbors are spying on her by listening to her through heating vents. Because of this, she has changed residences many times over the past 10 years. She looks peculiar and seems preoccupied by "voices talking in her head."

What is schizophrenia?

A chronic debilitating mental disorder characterized by disturbed thought, speech, and behavior; odd appearance; social withdrawal; poor grooming; abnormal affect (flat, blunted, or inappropriate)

Is the patient oriented, and how is her memory?

Usually well oriented to person, place, and time; intact memory

Is the patient in touch with reality?

In the residual phase, yes; in the psychotic phase, no

How long must symptoms be present for the DSM-IV-TR diagnosis?

1. 6 months of symptoms (prodromal, acute psychotic, and residual)
2. At least one period of actual psychosis within those 6 months
3. Impairment of occupational or social functioning must have occurred during this time period

Prodromal signs?

Quiet, passive or irritable, few friendships, avoids social activities, daydreams, somatic complaints, shows new interest in the occult, religion, or philosophy

What thought disorders are present during an acute psychotic episode?

Disorders of perception (e.g., hallucinations), disorders of thought content (e.g., delusions, ideas of reference, loss of ego boundaries), disorders of thought processes, disorders of form of thought

Residual signs and symptoms?

Flat affect, peculiar thinking and behavior, social withdrawal

What are hallucinations?

False sensory perceptions (e.g., hearing voices when alone in a room, smelling nonexistent odors)

What types of hallucinations are most common?

Auditory; visual, tactile, gustatory, olfactory, and cenesthetic (visceral sensation) hallucinations are less commonly seen

What are delusions?

False beliefs that are not corrrectable by reason or logic and are not based on simple ignorance or shared by a culture or subculture (e.g., the unrealistic idea of being followed by the FBI)

What types of delusions are most common?

Delusions of persecution (see above)

What is loss of ego boundaries?

The patient feels she is "merged" into others. She does not know where her mind and body end and those of others begin.

What are ideas of reference?

The patient believes that other people or the media are referring to her when they are not.

What are the disorders of thought processes?

Illogical ideas, thought blocking (abrupt halt in the train of thinking, often because of hallucinations), deficiencies in thought or content of speech, impaired abstraction ability, neologisms (making up new words; e.g., the patient refers to the doctor as a "medicrologist")

What are the disorders of form of thought?

Incoherence, word salad (unrelated combinations of words or phrases), loose associations (ideas shift from one subject to another in an unrelated fashion), paucity of speech, and echolalia (parroting a word just spoken by someone else)

What are the five subtypes of schizophrenia?

1. **Disorganized** (was called **hebephrenic**): disinhibited; poor organization, personal appearance, and grooming; inappropriate emotional responses; age of onset before 25 years
2. **Catatonic:** bizarre posturing (waxy flexibility) or extreme excitability, rare since introduction of antipsychotics
3. **Paranoid:** delusions of persecution; older age of onset and better functioning than other subtypes
4. **Undifferentiated:** characteristics of more than one subtype; most common type
5. **Residual:** has had one schizophrenic episode and subsequently shows residual symptoms but no psychotic symptoms

What are negative (deficit) symptoms?

Symptoms characterized by loss of function (e.g., flattened affect, thought blocking, cognitive disturbances, poor grooming, lack of motivation, social withdrawal, poor speech content); these respond better to atypical agents than to traditional antipsychotics

What are positive (productive) symptoms?

Symptoms characterized by "excessive" function (e.g., hallucinations, agitation, strange behavior, delusions, talkativeness); these respond both to atypical and traditional antipsychotics

In a research context, what physiologic measures are abnormal in schizophrenia?

Electroencephalogram (EEG) shows decreased alpha waves, increased theta and delta waves, and epileptiform activity

Eye movements (e.g., poor smooth visual pursuit) are abnormal in 50%-80% of patients as well as in unaffected relatives

Neuroendocrinology (e.g., decreased luteinizing hormone and follicle-stimulating hormone, and abnormal regulation of cortisol as demonstrated by a positive dexamethasone suppression test) in some patients

Laboratory tests may show elevated levels of homovanillic acid, a metabolite of dopamine, in body fluids

DDX

Medical illnesses that mimic schizophrenia?	Temporal lobe epilepsy, neurologic disease or trauma, poisoning, endocrine disorders
Psychiatric illnesses that mimic schizophrenia?	Brief psychotic disorder, schizophreniform disorder, schizoaffective disorder, manic phase of bipolar disorder, delusional disorder, schizoid and schizotypal personality disorders (see Chapters 9 and 20).
Other disorders that mimic schizophrenia?	Substance abuse, particularly amphetamines and hallucinogens (associated more commonly with visual and tactile rather than auditory hallucinations) [see Chapter 7]

OCCURRENCE

Risk for relatives of patients?	50% for monozygotic twins of schizophrenic persons 40% for those with two parents with schizophrenia 12% for first-degree relatives (child, sibling) of schizophrenic persons 1% for the general population
Age of onset in men versus women?	Peak for men, 15–25 years of age; for women, 25–35; in 90% of patients onset is at 15–45 years of age

Gender and race differences?	Equal prevalence in men and women and in all ethnic groups and cultures studied

ETIOLOGY

Brain pathology?	Decreased size of amygdala, hippocampus, and parahippocampal gyrus; movement problems implicate the basal ganglia; lateral and third ventricle enlargement; abnormal cerebral symmetry; changes in brain density; abnormalities of the frontal lobes as evidenced by decreased use of glucose in the prefrontal cortex on PET scans
Social/environmental factors?	None demonstrated to have causal relationship Internal or external stress may shorten time to onset or increase severity of symptoms (the "stress diathesis model")
What is the downward drift hypothesis?	People with schizophrenia are found more in low socioeconomic groups because they tend to drift down the socioeconomic scale as a result of their social deficits.
What is the dopamine hypothesis?	Schizophrenia results from excessive dopaminergic activity (e.g., excessive number of dopamine receptors, excessive concentration of dopamine, or hypersensitivity of receptors to dopamine).
Other neurotransmitters implicated?	**Serotonin** hyperactivity is implicated because hallucinogens that increase serotonin levels cause psychotic symptoms and because most effective atypical antipsychotics have antiserotonergic$_2$ (5-HT$_2$) activity. **Norepinephrine** hyperactivity is implicated, particularly in paranoid schizophrenia. **GABA** is implicated because patients show loss of GABA-ergic neurons in the hippocampus.

Glutamate is implicated because antagonists and agonists of glutamate receptors increase and decrease, respectively, some symptoms of schizophrenia.

TREATMENT

Pharmacologic treatment?

"Traditional" antipsychotics [dopamine$_2$ (D_2)-receptor antagonists] and atypical antipsychotic agents. Atypicals have recently become first-line agents.

Psychological treatment?

Individual, family, and group psychotherapy are useful for long-term support and to maintain compliance with drug regimen

What are the "traditional" antipsychotic agents?
  Low-potency agents?

Table 8–1

Agent	Oral Dose (mg/day)	Special Clinical Uses
Thioridazine (Mellaril)	200–600	Depression with intense anxiety or agitation
Chlorpromazine (Thorazine)	100–800	To treat nausea and vomiting, hiccups

  High-potency agents?

Table 8–2

Agent	Oral Dose (mg/day)	Special Clinical Uses
Haloperidol (Haldol)	2–20	Psychosis secondary to organic syndromes; Tourette disorder; available in long-acting (deconoate) form
Perphenazine (Trilafon)	8–64	To treat nausea and vomiting
Pimozide (Orap)	1–10	Tourette disorder, body dysmorphic disorder
Trifluoperazine (Stelazine)	4–20	Nonpsychotic anxiety (up to 12 weeks)
Fluphenazine (Prolixin)	2–15	Available in deconoate form

How do traditional antipsychotics work?

By blocking central D_2 receptors

| **How effective are traditional antipsychotics?** | Significant improvement is seen in 70% of patients (25% of these improve as a result of the placebo effect); they are particularly effective against positive symptoms |

What are the atypical antipsychotics?

Table 8–3

Agent	Oral Dose (mg/day)	Special Clinical Uses
Clozapine (Clozaril)	300–900	Particulary effective for negative, chronic, and refractory symptoms
Risperidone (Risperdal)	4–16	All others are useful for negative symptoms but have fewer neurological side effects than clozapine or the typical antipsychotics
Olanzapine (Zyprexa)	10–20	
Quetiapine (Seroquel)	50–800	
Ziprasidone (Geodon)	40–200	
Aripiprazole (Abilify)	10–30	

| **How do atypical antipsychotics work?** | **Clozapine** (Clozaril) acts on the serotonergic system and is also a D_1-, D_3-, and D_4-receptor antagonist. It is less likely to cause tardive dyskinesia, neuroleptic malignant syndrome, and parkinsonism. It does not cause extrapyramidal effects or dystonia. |
| | **Risperidone** (Risperdal), Olanzapine (Zyprexa), quetiapine (Seroquel), ziprasidone (Geodon), and aripiprazole (Abilify) also have antiserotonergic- as well as antidopaminergic-receptor activity and fewer neurologic side effects. |

Side effects of the antipsychotics?	**Low-potency antipsychotics** have mainly anticholinergic side effects.
	High-potency antipsychotics have mainly neurologic side effects.
	Clozapine and other atypicals are more likely to cause agranulocytosis, seizures, and anticholinergic side effects than are traditional agents.

Peripheral and central anticholinergic side effects?	**Peripheral effects** include dry mouth, blurred vision, constipation, and urinary retention. **Central effects** include severe agitation and confusion.
Treatment of anticholinergic side effects?	**Peripheral effects** are treated with salivary stimulants for dry mouth, hydration for urinary hesitancy, stool softeners for constipation, and physostigmine eye drops for blurred vision. **Central effects** are treated with physostigmine (Antilirium, 1–2 mg IM or IV) repeated in 30 minutes.
Neurologic side effects?	**Parkinsonian effects:** resting ("pill rolling") tremor, akinesia, and rigidity **Acute dystonia:** slow, prolonged muscular spasms, most common in men younger than age 40 years **Akathisia:** subjective feeling of motor restlessness **Neuroleptic malignant syndrome:** high fever, sweating, confusion, increased blood pressure and pulse, muscular rigidity, high creatine phosphokinase concentration, and renal failure. Twenty percent mortality rate, more common in men, and more common early in the treatment program **Tardive dyskinesia:** writhing (choreathetoid) movements of tongue, head, face, and mouth, more common in older women, usually occurs after 6 months of antipsychotic treatment
Treatment of parkinsonian effects?	Reduce dose of antipsychotic agent **Anticholinergic agents:** Amantadine (Symmetrel; 100–200 mg/day), benztropine (Cogentin; 1–4 mg/day), trihexyphenidyl (Artane; 2–5 mg/day), or diphenhydramine (Benadryl; 25–50 mg/day)
Treatment of neuroleptic malignant syndrome?	This is a medical emergency! Immediately discontinue antipsychotic

agents. Supportive medical treatment includes hypothermia and hydration, dantrolene (Dantrium; up to 10 mg/kg/day IV); bromocriptine (Parlodel) and amantadine (Symmetrel) are also useful.

Treatment of tardive dyskinesia?

Discontinue traditional antipsychotic and substitute an atypical agent. Treatments that have been used with modest success include benzodiazepines, propranolol, and cholinomimetics (e.g., choline chloride).

Other side effects of antipsychotics?

1. **Weight gain** and **sedation,** especially with atypical agents; possibly Type II diabetes mellitus
2. **Circulatory:** electrocardiogram abnormalities, orthostatic hypotension
3. **Endocrine:** increased prolactin resulting in gynecomastia, galactorrhea, impotence, amenorrhea, decreased libido
4. **Hematologic:** leukopenia, agranulocytosis (deficiency in some white blood cells, particularly polymorphonuclear leukocytes), especially with clozapine
5. **Hepatic:** jaundice, elevated liver enzymes
6. **Dermatologic:** photosensitivity, skin eruptions, blue-gray skin discoloration with chlorpromazine
7. **Ophthalmologic:** irreversible retinal pigmentation from thioridazine, deposits in lens and cornea from chlorpromazine

Treatment for noncompliant patients?

Fluphenazine (Prolixin) decanoate and haloperidol (Haldol) decanoate (long-acting injectable depot forms) administered intramuscularly every 4 weeks

COURSE AND PROGNOSIS

What indicates that a patient is going to have a psychotic episode?

Increasing agitation, depression, and insomnia

Usual course of the illness?

Repeated psychotic episodes; chronic, downhill course; often stabilizes in midlife

What happens after an acute psychotic episode is over?

Depression in 50% of patients; suicide attempts may occur

Prognosis?

Chronic, lifelong impairment; better prognosis if patient has mood symptoms, is older at onset, is married or has social relationships, is female, has good employment history, has positive symptoms, and has had few relapses

9   Other Psychotic Disorders

What five disorders other than schizophrenia present with psychotic symptoms?

1. Brief psychotic disorder
2. Schizophreniform disorder
3. Schizoaffective disorder
4. Delusional disorder
5. Shared psychotic disorder (folie à deux)

What other disorders are included in the differential diagnoses of schizophrenia?

Manic phase of bipolar disorder (see Chapter 10)

Schizotypal, schizoid, paranoid, and borderline personality disorders (see Chapter 20)

Delirium and dementia (see Chapter 6)

Psychotic disorder due to a general medical condition

Substance-induced psychotic disorder

BRIEF PSYCHOTIC DISORDER

Typical patient?

A 27-year-old woman whose brother died recently of AIDS is brought by relatives to the hospital. They claim that over the past week she has begun to behave strangely and to claim that she hears her brother "talking to her inside her head."

Characteristics?

Psychotic and residual symptoms lasting at least 1 day but less than 1 month; more common in patients with concomitant borderline and histrionic personality disorders than in the general population

How does it compare with schizophrenia?

Duration of symptoms is shorter than in schizophrenia

Symptoms often follow exposure to a psychosocial stressor; there may be no stressor in schizophrenia

Patient was relatively normal in the
premorbid period; the schizophrenic
Patient usually shows premorbid
symptoms such as withdrawal, strange
behavior, and odd beliefs
No family history of schizophrenia

Treatment?   Short hospital stay, structure, support and
reassurance
Antipsychotic medication
Benzodiazepines
Psychotherapy for dealing with the
stressful precipitating event (if
present)

Prognosis?   50%–80% recover completely; 20%–50%
may ultimately be diagnosed with
schizophrenia or a mood disorder

SCHIZOPHRENIFORM DISORDER

Typical patient?   A 26-year-old man with no previous
history of psychiatric illness is brought to
the emergency room by his girlfriend.
She tells you that about 3 months ago, he
suddenly began to show bizarre behavior,
often seemed preoccupied as though he
was listening to something, and showed
abrupt mood changes.

Characteristics?   Two or more psychotic symptoms lasting
at least 1 month but less than 6 months

**How does it compare with
schizophrenia?**   Duration of symptoms is shorter than in
schizophrenia
Impairment of social or occupational
functioning are not necessary for the
diagnosis

Treatment?   Hospitalization
Antipsychotic medication
Psychotherapy to deal with the
experience of having had a psychotic
episode

Prognosis?   33% recover completely; 66% progress to
schizoaffective disorder or
schizophrenia

SCHIZOAFFECTIVE DISORDER

Typical patient?

A 35-year-old man with a history of psychotic symptoms and severe depression has never held a job for more than 3 months. He is successfully treated for his depressive symptoms but remains withdrawn and psychotic.

Characteristics?

Fits the criteria for both mood disorder and schizophrenia; chronic impairment in functioning between episodes

How does it compare with schizophrenia?

In schizoaffective disorder, the criteria for mania or depression as well as for schizophrenia are met

Treatment?

Hospitalization
Antidepressants, mood stabilizers, and electroconvulsive therapy; antipsychotic agents are used for psychotic episodes or may be the primary treatment if mood stabilizers are ineffective

Prognosis?

Better than for schizophrenia, worse than for mood disorder; chronic and lifelong

DELUSIONAL DISORDER

Typical patient?

A 55-year-old patient tells you that his neighbor has been plotting for years to get him arrested by listening in on all of his phone conversations. The patient is married and has been in the same job for 25 years.

Characteristics?

A rare disorder characterized by a fixed, nonbizarre delusional system (often paranoid); few if any other thought disorders; more common in immigrants, the hearing impaired, and patients older than 40 years of age

How does it compare with schizophrenia?

Content of delusions is unlikely but not impossible (e.g., my neighbor wants to get me into trouble with the health department); in schizophrenia, content of delusions is bizarre (e.g., "my neighbor told the devil to hurt me")

Patient rarely has other thought disorders; delusional thinking is circumscribed, not affecting other areas of the patient's life; because of many thought problems, social function is abnormal in schizophrenia

Treatment?

Psychotherapy to gain the patient's trust

Trial of pimozide (Orap) (particularly for somatic delusions) or haloperidol (Haldol), although antipsychotics are often not effective

Prognosis?

50% recover, 30% remain the same, 20% show decreased symptoms; younger age at onset, sudden onset, and presence of precipitating factors are associated with a good prognosis

SHARED PSYCHOTIC DISORDER (FOLIE À DEUX)

Typical patient?

A 20-year-old woman whose psychotic husband believes that the landlord is trying to poison him now begins to believe the same thing.

Characteristics?

Development of delusional symptoms in a person in a close relationship with another person (usually a spouse or other family member) who already has similar delusional symptoms (the inducer); more common in women and in people from lower socioeconomic groups

How does it compare with schizophrenia?

The psychotic symptoms occur only after exposure to the inducer; in schizophrenia, there is no inducer

Treatment?

Remove the patient from the influence of the inducer

Social support and psychotherapy

Antipsychotic medication

Prognosis?

10%–40% of cases resolve with separation from the inducer; such separation may be impractical if the inducer is a family member.

OTHER DISORDERS THAT MAY BE CONFUSED WITH SCHIZOPHRENIA

How does schizoid personality disorder compare with schizophrenia?

In both conditions there is social withdrawal; however, there is no psychosis in schizoid personality disorder

How does schizotypal personality disorder compare with schizophrenia?

In both conditions there are bizarre behavior and peculiar thought patterns, such as magical thinking (e.g., the idea that wishing can make something happen); however, in schizotypal personality disorder there is no frank psychosis.

How does delirium compare with schizophrenia?

In both conditions there are hallucinations; however, in delirium the hallucinations are often visual and changeable and in schizophrenia they are often auditory and relatively constant.

Consciousness is clouded in delirium and normal in schizophrenia.

Delirium occurs in the context of an acute medical problem.

How does the manic phase of bipolar disorder compare with schizophrenia?

In both conditions there may be psychotic symptoms, such as delusions.

In mania there is an obvious elevation of mood, hyperactivity, and rapid speech; mood changes in schizophrenia are inconsistent and mood incongruent.

In mania, there is little or no impairment in social functioning between episodes; in schizophrenia, there is marked impairment in social functioning in the residual phase.

Mood Disorders

OVERVIEW

What are the mood (or affective) disorders?	Disorders with a primary disturbance in mood or emotional state causing subjective distress and occupational or social problems
DSM-IV-TR categories of mood disorders?	Major depressive disorder, bipolar I disorder, bipolar II disorder, dysthymic disorder, cyclothymic disorder, mood disorder due to a general medical condition, substance-induced mood disorder, and adjustment disorder with depressed mood
Biologic etiology?	Altered neurotransmitter activity, primarily serotonin and norepinephrine Abnormalities of the limbic hypothalamic-pituitary-adrenal axis Altered sleep cycle
Psychosocial etiology of depression?	Loss of a parent in childhood Social loss during adult life (such as loss of a spouse) Negative interpretation of life events, low self-esteem, and loss of hope

MAJOR DEPRESSIVE DISORDER

CHARACTERISTICS

Typical patient?	A 40-year-old woman who has lost interest in her work and social life and lacks energy, motivation, and appetite (she has lost weight), admits to thoughts of suicide. She tells you that although she feels hopeless and helpless most of the time, she seems to feel a bit better in the evening than in the morning (diurnal variation in symptoms).

What is it?

Episodes of severely depressed mood resulting in loss of pleasure and interest in usual activities

Do psychotic symptoms occur in major depressive disorder?

Sometimes (depression with psychotic features), but paranoid delusions or auditory hallucinations are uncommon

How common are somatic symptoms?

They are common and range from mild hypochondriasis to somatic delusions (e.g., "I feel like I am rotting inside.").

What is anhedonia?

Loss of pleasure in most or all activities and inability to respond to pleasurable stimuli seen in depression with melancholic features

What does the mnemonic Sig:E Caps mean?

S Sleep (e.g., insomnia or early-morning awakening)
I Interest (e.g., decreased motivation and interest in activities)
G Guilt (e.g., excessive self-blame)
E Energy (e.g., loss of vigor is common)
C Concentration (e.g., difficulty paying attention and memory disturbances)
A Appetite (e.g., typically decreased appetite for food and sex)
P Psychomotor activity (e.g., typically decreased, particularly in the elderly; agitation may also occur)
S Suicidal ideation (e.g., thoughts of self-destruction are often present)

Are patients aware that they are depressed?

Up to 50% of depressed patients seem unaware of or may deny depression (i.e., "masked" depression) even though symptoms (often vague and somatic) are present.

What is the patient like between episodes of depression?

Usually normal

How often do episodes of depression occur?

Five or six episodes over a 20-year period; frequency and length of episodes increase with age

DDX

Medical conditions associated with depression?	1. Cancers, particularly pancreatic or other abdominal cancers, may present initially as depression
	2. Renal and cardiopulmonary diseases
	3. Viral illnesses (e.g., pneumonia, influenza, mononucleosis, AIDS)
	4. Neurologic illnesses [e.g., Parkinson disease, multiple sclerosis, dementia, stroke (particularly left frontal)]
	5. Nutritional deficiency
	6. Endocrine abnormalities, particularly thyroid dysfunction
	7. Prescription drugs (e.g., reserpine, propranolol, steroids, methyldopa)
Psychiatric conditions associated with depression?	Drug and alcohol abuse and withdrawal; particularly abuse of sedative drugs and withdrawal from stimulant drugs
	Anxiety disorders
	Schizophrenia (particularly after an acute psychotic episode)
	Somatoform disorders

OCCURRENCE

Gender differences?	Lifetime prevalence of 5%–12% for men and 10%–20% for women
Ethnic differences?	None
Association with education, marital state, income?	None

TREATMENT

Pharmacologic treatments?	Heterocyclic antidepressants, selective serotonin reuptake inhibitors (SSRIs), monoamine oxidase inhibitors (MAOIs), other antidepressants, and mood stabilizers

Table 10–1
Antidepressant Agents

Classification	Agent	Dose (mg/day)	Special Clinical Uses
Heterocyclics	Amitriptyline (Elavil)	75–300	Depression with insomnia
	Clomipramine (Anafranil)	100–250	Obsessive–compulsive disorder
	Desipramine (Norpramin, Pertofrane)	75–300	Depression in the elderly, anorexia nervosa, bulimia
	Doxepin (Adapin, Sinequan)	150–300	Generalized anxiety disorder, peptic ulcer disease
	Imipramine (Tofranil)	150–300	Panic disorder with agoraphobia, enuresis, anorexia nervosa, bulimia
	Maprotiline (Ludiomil)	150–225	Anxiety with depressive features
	Nortriptyline (Aventyl, Pamelor)	50–150	Depression in cardiac patients and the elderly
SSRIs	Fluoxetine (Prozac, Sarafem, Prozac weekly)	20–80	Obsessive–compulsive disorder (OCD), premature ejaculation, panic disorder, premenstrual dysphoric disorder (Sarafem), paraphilias, hyphochondriasis, social phobia, chronic pain, PTSD, migraine headaches, bulimia
	Paroxetine (Paxil)	20–60	Same as fluoxetine
	Sertraline (Zoloft)	50–200	Same as fluoxetine
	Fluvoxamine (Luvox)	100–300	OCD
	Citalopram (Celexa)	20–60	Same as fluoxetine
	Escitalopram (Lexapro)	10–20	Same as fluoxetine
MAOIs	Phenelzine (Nardil)	60–90	Atypical depression, panic disorder, eating disorders, pain disorders, social phobia
	Tranylcypromine (Parnate)	20–60	Same as phenelzine
Other anti- depressants	Amoxapine (Asendin)	200–400	Depression with psychotic features
	Bupropion (Wellbutrin, Wellbutrin SR, Zyban)	200–450 200–400,[a] 150–300,[b]	Intolerance of other antidepressants, refractory depression, smoking cessation (Zyban), seasonal affective disorder, SSRI-induced sexual dysfunction, adult ADHD

Continues

Table 10–1 *(continued)*
Antidepressant Agents

Classification	Agent	Dose (mg/day)	Special Clinical Uses
	Nefazodone (Serzone)	300–600	Intolerance of other antidepressants
	Mirtazapine (Remeron)	15–25	Refractory depression (first alpha-2 antagonist indicated for depression, may increase appetite), insomnia
	Trazodone (Desyrel)	200–600	Insomnia
	Venlafaxine (Effexor, Effexor XR)		Refractory depression (fastest action works within 10 days), generalized anxiety disorder

[a]Dose for Wellbutrin SR.
[b]Dose for Zyban.

Which agents are most commonly used?	Although heterocyclics used to be the mainstay of treatment, the SSRIs, such as fluoxetine, are now used as first-line drugs because they have more tolerable side effects.
Which agents have the most efficacy?	All antidepressants have similar efficacy
How long do antidepressants take to work?	All take at least 3-6 weeks to work
Can combinations of antidepressants be used?	Combinations of heterocyclic antidepressant agents with MAOIs can be used with extreme caution. Lithium or thyroid hormone (T_3) may be used to augment the efficacy of antidepressants. Combinations of antipsychotics and antidepressants may be used in patients who have depression with psychotic features.
Five major side effects of the heterocyclics?	1. Sedation 2. Anticholinergic effects 3. Cardiovascular effects such as orthostatic hypotension 4. Weight gain 5. Dangerous in overdose

The major side effect of the MAOIs?

Hypertensive crisis with the ingestion of tyramine-rich foods (beer, wine, broad beans, aged cheese, beef or chicken liver, orange pulp, smoked or pickled meats or fish), sympathomimetic drugs, dangerous in overdose

The major side effects of the SSRIs?

Activation and insomnia (particularly with fluoxetine); sexual problems, particularly delayed orgasm; fewer anticholinergic and cardiovascular side effects than other antidepressants; are safer in overdose; may cause minor weight loss initially

What is electroconvulsive therapy (ECT)?

ECT involves the induction of a generalized seizure lasting 25 to 60 seconds by passing a current of electricity across the brain.

Major indication for ECT?

Major depressive disorder refractory to antidepressants, or when rapid resolution of symptoms is imperative because of suicide risk

How is ECT administered?

Premedication (atropine 0.6–1.2 mg IM) followed by general anesthesia [sodium methohexital (Brevital): 40–100 mg IV] and a muscle relaxant [succinylcholine (Anectine): 30–80 mg IV] are given before seizure induction.

How is a seizure induced in unilateral, bifrontal, and bilateral ECT?

In unilateral ECT, two electrodes are placed on the nondominant hemisphere, one on the frontotemporal area and the other in the parietal area.
In bifrontal ECT, one electrode is placed at the end of each eyebrow.
In bilateral ECT, one electrode is placed on each temple.

What is the difference between unilateral, bifrontal, and bilateral ECT?

Compared with the traditional bilateral ECT, there are fewer side effects but less efficacy with bifrontal and unilateral ECT.

How many ECT treatments are given?

Eight treatments over a 2- to 3-week period

Major adverse effect of ECT?	Amnesia (usually retrograde), which usually remits within 6 months
Major absolute contraindications for ECT?	Increased intracranial pressure or recent (within 2 weeks) myocardial infarction
How is improvement maintained after ECT?	Antidepressant agent or maintenance outpatient ECT once or twice per month
What psychological treatments are used for depression?	Psychoanalytically-oriented, interpersonal, family, behavior, and cognitive therapy (see Chapter 25)
What is the most effective treatment?	Psychological treatment used in conjunction with medication is more beneficial than either treatment alone.
What are the three major reasons for hospitalizing a depressed patient?	1. High suicide risk (e.g., has a ready means and plan for suicide, such as a gun and a chosen time and place) 2. Concomitant use of alcohol or other substance of abuse 3. Psychotic symptoms

PROGNOSIS

How long does an episode of depression last?	If untreated, depression is self-limiting and lasts from 6 to 12 months.
What percentage of depressed patients seek treatment for their symptoms?	About 25%
What percentage of patients can be treated successfully?	About 75%; 15% of patients with major depressive disorder eventually commit suicide.
When in the illness is the risk of suicide highest for patients?	Frequently, patients with severe depression do not have the energy to commit suicide; the risk of suicide increases as depression lifts and energy returns with treatment
What are the top five risks for suicide?	1. Serious prior suicide attempt 2. Older age

3. Substance abuse or dependence
4. History of rage and violent behavior
5. Male gender

What are eight other risk factors for suicide?

1. Unmarried status
2. White race
3. Family history of suicide
4. Psychotic symptoms
5. Chronic illness
6. Jewish or Protestant religion
7. Economic recession or depression
8. Low job satisfaction

BIPOLAR DISORDER

CHARACTERISTICS

Typical patient during a manic episode?

A 30-year-old man who is grandiose, distractible, and delusional (he thinks he receives mental messages from Tom Cruise) has been brought to the emergency room. When stopped by police because he was running down the street naked (disinhibited with impaired judgment), he became very irritable and physically resisted the officers' attempts to restrain him (assaultive).

What mood symptoms are present?

Episodes of elevated mood and major depression

What is bipolar I disorder?

Episodes of both mania (very elevated mood) and major depression

What is bipolar II disorder?

Episodes of both hypomania (elevated mood not as severe as in mania) and major depression

Which phase usually comes first?

The depressed phase; the first manic or hypomanic episode usually occurs before age 30 years

How long does a manic episode last?

If untreated, about 3 months

What does the depressed phase of bipolar disorder look like?

Like depression in major depressive disorder; the first episode may show some differences.

| **What characterizes the first depressive episode in a patient who will ultimately show mania?** | Psychotic symptoms, psychomotor retardation, mania or hypomania after antidepressant drug therapy, and postpartum depression |

| **What diagnosis is given to a person who shows only mania?** | Bipolar disorder (there is no such thing as pure manic disorder; there will eventually be a depressive episode) |

| **DDx?** | Schizophrenia, schizoaffective disorder, substance abuse, delirium, cyclothymic disorder |

OCCURRENCE

| **Risk for relatives of patients?** | 75% for monozygotic twins of patients with bipolar disorder
60% for those with two parents with bipolar disorder
20% for first-degree relatives (brother, father) of patients with bipolar disorder
1% for the general population |

| **Gender differences?** | Occurs equally in men and women |

| **Ethnic differences?** | None; however, because of limited access to health care, mood disorders, particularly bipolar disorder in poor black and Hispanic patients, may progress to a point at which their illness is misdiagnosed as schizophrenia rather than bipolar disorder |

Table 10–2
Mood Stabilizers

Agent	Dose (mg/day)
Lithium [Eskalith, Eskalith SR (controlled-release)]	900–1800 (titrated to a blood level of 0.8–1.2 mEq/L, although levels of 0.6–0.8 mEq/L may be adequate)
Carbamazepine (Tegretol)	400–1000 (titrated to a blood level of 4–12 μg/mL)
Valproic acid (Depakene) and divalproex [Depakote (more slowly absorbed form of valproic acid)]	500–1500 (titrated to a blood level of 50–100 μg/mL)
Oxcarbazepine (Trileptal)	300–1200 (titrated to a blood level of 4–12 μg/mL)

TREATMENT

What is the drug of choice for treating bipolar disorder?	Lithium
What two other uses does lithium have?	1. To control aggressive behavior 2. To enhance the activity of tricyclic antidepressants
What are the major adverse effects of lithium?	First trimester congenital abnormalities (especially Ebstein's anomaly, a cardiac malformation), tremor, renal dysfunction, cardiac conduction problems, hypothyroidism, acne, gastric distress, mild cognitive impairment
What other drugs are used to treat bipolar disorder?	Anticonvulsants, such as carbamazepine (Tegretol) and valproic acid [Depakene or divalproex (Depakote), and oxcarbazepine (Trileptal)]; carbamazepine is used also in trigeminal neuralgia and valproic acid is used also in treating bipolar symptoms resulting from a cognitive disorder. Anticonvulsants are particularly useful in rapid cycling bipolar disorder (more than four episodes yearly) and mixed episodes (mixed manic and depressive features)
What are the major adverse effects of carbamazepine?	Aplastic anemia, agranulocytosis, sedation, dizziness, ataxia, congenital anomalies
What are the major adverse effects of valproic acid and divalproex?	Gastrointestinal symptoms, liver problems, congenital neural tube defects, alopecia, weight gain
What are the major side effects of oxcarbazepine?	Dizziness, ataxia, visual disturbances, no blood dyscrasias or autoinduction
What newer drugs have mood stabilizing action?	Anticonvulsants like lamotrigine (Lamictal), gabapentin (Neurontin), tiagabine (Gabitril), and topiramate (Topamax)

PROGNOSIS

How do the prognoses of the two major mood disorders compare?	Bipolar disorder has a worse prognosis than major depressive disorder.

| How does bipolar disorder progress? | The period of time between manic episodes (generally 6–9 months) becomes shorter as bipolar illness progresses. |

MINOR MOOD DISORDERS: DYSTHYMIC AND CYCLOTHYMIC DISORDERS

CHARACTERISTICS

Typical dysthymic patient?	A 23-year-old woman has been "down in the dumps" since her junior year in college two years ago. Fellow students describe her as demanding and complaining, and she seems resistant to attempts at psychotherapy.
Typical cyclothymic patient?	A 30-year-old man seems unusually energetic and optimistic (an "up," or hypomanic period) for the last three months. Previously, he had been described as glum and moody.
What are dysthymic and cyclothymic disorders?	Dysthymic disorder involves mild or moderate depression most of the time with no discrete episodes. Cyclothymic disorder involves episodes of hypomania as well as mild or moderate depression.
How long must symptoms be present to make a diagnosis?	For both disorders, the symptoms must have been present for at least 2 years.

DDX

| **What is the most common differential diagnosis for dysthymic disorder?** | Bereavement or adjustment disorder with depressed mood; in contrast to dysthymic disorder, here, a clearly identifiable life stress precipitated the depressive symptoms, which remit over time |
| **What two psychiatric conditions are most closely associated with these disorders?** | Substance abuse [particularly of central nervous system (CNS) depressants may resemble dysthymia; patients taking stimulants may look hypomanic] and major depressive disorder (the residual phase is characterized by dysthymic disorder in some patients, so-called "double depression") |

What is the major difference between major depressive disorder and dysthymia?	Major depressive disorder is episodic and severe and results in severely impaired social and occupational functioning, whereas dysthymic disorder is nonepisodic, chronic, less severe, results in mild, moderate, or severe impairment in functioning, and is never associated with psychosis.

OCCURRENCE

How common is dysthymic disorder?	About 3% to 5% of the population
How common is cyclothymic disorder?	Less than 1% of the population
What is the most common age of onset?	Half of patients have symptoms of dysthymic disorder before age 25 years (early-onset type). The most common age of onset for cyclothymic disorder is 15–25 years.
Gender differences?	Dysthymic disorder is two to three times more common in women; cyclothymic disorder is equal in both.

ETIOLOGY

What two factors have been identified in the etiology of dysthymic disorder?	Loss of a close relative and chronic medical illness in childhood

TREATMENT

What are the two most effective psychological treatment modalities for dysthymic disorder?	Cognitive therapy and insight-oriented psychotherapy; cognitive therapy is a behavioral method of short-term psychotherapy (up to 25 weeks) in which the patient's distorted, negative thinking is replaced with self-enhancing thoughts (see Chapters 24 and 25)
Is pharmacotherapy useful in dysthymic disorder?	Although not believed in the past to be effective in this condition, antidepressants are now commonly used. The MAOIs are more effective than heterocyclic agents when there is a large anxiety component,

and SSRIs appear to be more effective than both.

What is the primary treatment for cyclothymic disorder?	Antimanic agents in doses similar to those used for bipolar disorder (lithium in smaller doses)

PROGNOSIS

For dysthymic disorder?	20% of patients go on to major depressive disorder and 20% go on to bipolar disorder (I or II); at least 25% retain similar symptoms throughout life
For cyclothymic disorder?	Chronic and lifelong; 33% eventually are diagnosed with bipolar disorder

11   Anxiety Disorders

OVERVIEW

What are the anxiety disorders?	A group of mental disorders characterized by the subjective and physiologic manifestations of fear
What distinguishes anxiety from fear?	In anxiety, the individual experiences apprehension, but, in contrast to fear, the source of the danger is not known, not recognized, or inadequate to account for the symptoms.
What are the physical manifestations of anxiety?	Similar to those of fear, including sweating, shakiness, dizziness, palpitations (subjective experiences of tachycardia), mydriasis (pupil dilation), syncope, tingling in the extremities, perioral loss of sensation, tremor, gastrointestinal disturbances such as diarrhea, and urinary urgency and frequency
What medical conditions are associated with symptoms of anxiety?	Excessive caffeine intake, substance abuse, vitamin B_{12} deficiency, hyperthyroidism, hypoglycemia, cardiac arrhythmias, mitral valve prolapse, and pheochromocytoma (an adrenal medullary tumor)
Etiology?	Unknown. Psychosocial, biologic, and genetic factors may contribute. Neurotransmitters involved include γ-aminobutyric acid (GABA; decreased activity), norepinephrine (increased activity), and serotonin (decreased activity).
What are the six major DSM-IV classifications of anxiety disorders?	1. Panic disorder 2. Phobias 3. Obsessive-compulsive disorder (OCD) 4. Generalized anxiety disorder (GAD) 5. Posttraumatic stress disorder (PTSD) and acute stress disorder (ASD)

6. Anxiety disorder not otherwise specified (NOS); persistent anxiety symptoms that do not meet the full criteria for another anxiety disorder

What are two other classifications of anxiety disorders?

1. Anxiety disorder due to a general medical condition
2. Substance-induced anxiety disorder

PANIC DISORDER (WITH OR WITHOUT AGORAPHOBIA)

CHARACTERISTICS

Typical patient?

A 26-year-old, apparently healthy woman comes to the ER terrified, feeling impending doom and convinced that she is having a heart attack.

What is it?

Episodic panic attacks; i.e., periods of anxiety symptoms that have a sudden onset and increase in intensity over an approximately 10-minute period

How often do panic attacks occur and how long do they last?

They occur about twice weekly and last about 30 minutes. Between attacks the patient fears having another attack (anticipatory anxiety).

What is panic disorder with agoraphobia?

Panic attacks that are triggered by exposure to an open place (e.g., when the patient goes outside of his or her home alone) or to a situation where escape or help is unavailable

DDX

The symptoms of which medical condition most resemble those of panic disorder?

Myocardial infarction, because shortness of breath, chest discomfort, tachycardia, and sweating occur in both

Which psychological conditions are most closely associated with panic disorder?

Social or specific phobias, generalized anxiety disorder, depression, schizophrenia (just prior to a psychotic episode), malingering, hypochondriasis, and factitious disorder

For diagnostic purposes, how can a panic attack be induced in a panic disorder patient?	Attacks can be induced in the physician's office by IV administration of sodium lactate or by inhalation of CO_2 (breathing in and out of a paper bag)
What is the association between panic disorder and mitral valve prolapse?	Although these two conditions are associated, no causal relationship has been demonstrated.
What is the association between panic disorder and depression?	Depression is present in about 50% of panic disorder patients.
What childhood psychiatric disorder is associated with panic disorder?	Separation anxiety disorder

OCCURRENCE

What percentage of the population has panic disorder?	Panic disorder has a lifetime prevalence of 1.5–3.5%.
Is there a sex or age difference?	It is more common in women, and the mean age of onset is 25 years.
Genetic component?	Yes. First-degree relatives have a 4 to 7 times greater chance of also having panic disorder.
Social component?	Often, divorce or marital separation has occurred in the patient's recent past.

TREATMENT

First choice treatment for an acute attack?	Benzodiazepines
Most useful benzodiazepine?	Alprazolam (Xanax; 2–6 mg/day)
Major long-term pharmacologic treatment?	The antidepressants, particularly the selective serotonin reuptake inhibitors (SSRIs)
How long is pharmacologic treatment continued?	8–12 months, with gradual withdrawal

Most useful psychological treatments?	Systematic desensitization and cognitive therapy are useful adjuncts to pharmacotherapy.

PROGNOSIS

What is the course?	The condition has a chronic course with many recurrent episodes.
What percentage of patients relapse?	Up to 90% of patients relapse with discontinuation of medication.

PHOBIAS

CHARACTERISTICS

Typical patient?	She tries to avoid it, but a 32-year-old woman must give a brief work-related presentation. Although she knows all of the people in the small audience, she "freezes up" and is unable to give the talk.
What is specific phobia?	An irrational fear of certain specific things (e.g., animals, heights, needles), or situations (e.g., closed spaces, heights); because of the fear, the thing or situation is avoided
What is social phobia?	An exaggerated fear of social or environmental situations in which one could embarrass oneself in front of others (e.g., public speaking, using public restrooms, eating in a restaurant); because of the fear, the situation is avoided

DDX

Major differential diagnoses of specific phobia?	OCD, hypochondriasis, paranoid personality disorder, panic disorder, delusional disorder
Major differential diagnoses of social phobia?	Normal shyness, schizoid personality disorder, major depressive disorder, anorexia nervosa, bulimia nervosa

OCCURRENCE

How common is specific phobia?	Very common; specific phobia has a lifetime prevalence of 7%–11% in the population

How common is social phobia?	Has a lifetime prevalence of 3%–13% in the population

TREATMENT

Best treatment for specific phobia?	Systematic desensitization is most effective; hypnosis, family therapy, and psychotherapy are also useful. There is no effective pharmacologic treatment.
Best treatment for social phobia?	Pharmacologic treatment: 1. Antidepressants, primarily MAOIs (e.g., phenelzine) 2. β-adrenergic antagonists, such as propranolol (Inderal) [20–40 mg] or atenolol (Tenormin) [50–100 mg], are also useful, particularly for performance or test anxiety
What psychological treatments are useful in social phobia?	Assertiveness training and group therapy

PROGNOSIS

What happens to patients with specific or social phobias?	Secondary morbidity (e.g., school dropout, failure to marry, vocational impairment) is common.

OBSESSIVE-COMPULSIVE DISORDER (OCD)

CHARACTERISTICS

Typical patient?	Before he can go to sleep at night, a 35-year-old man must check the locks on his front door 10 times, and he often gets out of bed during the night to recheck the locks. He is often tired during the daytime because of this behavior.
What characterizes patients with OCD?	Recurrent intrusive thoughts, feelings, and images (obsessions), which cause anxiety that is relieved in part by performing repetitive actions (compulsions); most patients know that these thoughts and behaviors are irrational (i.e., they have insight)

Most common obsessions and compulsions?	Contamination (e.g., washing hands after touching objects), checking (door locks, gas jets), counting, and putting things in order
What evidence of neurologic abnormalities may be present?	Electroencephalographic (EEG) abnormalities; neuroendocrine and sleep studies show abnormalities similar to those seen in patients with depression (e.g., decreased REM latency)
What is the association between OCD and social factors?	OCD often begins after a stressful life event.

DDX

What conditions does OCD resemble?	Tourette disorder, obsessive-compulsive personality disorder
Most closely associated psychiatric condition?	In 20%–30% of patients with OCD, major depressive disorder also is present.

OCCURRENCE

How common is OCD?	Common; it occurs in 2%–3% of the population
At what age does it most commonly begin?	Most often in the third decade of life, but may begin in childhood
Genetic component?	There is a higher concordance rate in monozygotic than in dizygotic twins and in first-degree relatives of OCD patients.

TREATMENT

Most closely associated neurotransmitter?	Serotonin, based on the therapeutic success of the SSRIs and clomipramine (Anafronil) in treating OCD
Most useful pharmacologic treatments?	Fluoxetine (40–80 mg/day), fluvoxamine (Luvox) [100–300 mg/day], and other SSRIs; clomipramine (150–250 mg/day); all must be titrated slowly up to the effective dose
Most useful psychological treatments?	Behavior therapy (e.g., flooding and implosion; see Chapter 25)

Supportive psychotherapy (see Chapter 24)

PROGNOSIS

What percentage of patients improve with treatment?	One third of patients improve significantly and one half improve moderately; the remainder fail to improve or get worse.

GENERALIZED ANXIETY DISORDER

CHARACTERISTICS

Typical patient?	A 45-year-old woman comes in complaining of chronic diarrhea. She tells you that she has always been "nervous and high-strung."
Symptoms?	Persistent symptoms of "free-floating" anxiety, including hyperarousal lasting at least 6 months
What is free-floating anxiety?	Symptoms of anxiety that cannot be related to a specific person or situation
What are two closely associated psychiatric conditions?	1. Major depressive disorder 2. Dysthymic disorder

DDX

What other psychological conditions look like generalized anxiety disorder?	Other anxiety disorders, particularly panic disorder

OCCURRENCE

Is there a gender or age difference in its occurrence?	It is slightly more common in women (55%–60%) than in men (40%–45%) and, in 50% of patients, starts during childhood or adolescence.

TREATMENT

Most effective psychological treatments?	Cognitive and behavioral therapy

Most effective pharmacologic treatments?

Antianxiety agents, including:

1. Benzodiazepines, particularly those that have an intermediate length of action, because they work rapidly and last for a reasonably long time, but have less addiction potential than short-acting agents. Because benzodiazepines carry a high risk of dependence and addiction, they are used primarily for acute exacerbations of symptoms for weeks to months.
2. Buspirone (Bu Spar) [15–60 mg/day] is most useful for patients who have never been treated with or who cannot use benzodiazepines; it takes 2–3 weeks to work.

Antidepressants, including: venlafaxine (Effexor) and doxepin (Adapin or Sinequan)

Table 11–1
Antianxiety Agents

Classification	Agent (Duration)	Dose (mg/day)	Special Clinical Uses
Benzodiazepines	Lorazepam (Ativan) [short]	2–6	Psychotic agitation
	Oxazepam (Serax) [short]	30–120	Alcohol withdrawal
	Triazolam (Halcion) [short]	0.125–0.25	Insomnia
	Alprazolam (Xanax) [intermediate]	0.5–6	Antidepressant, panic disorder, social phobia
	Temazepam (Restoril) [intermediate]	15–30	Insomnia
	Chlordiazepoxide (Librium) [long]	15–100	Alcohol withdrawal
	Clonazepam (Klonopin) [long]	0.5–4	Seizures, mania, social phobia, panic disorder
	Diazepam (Valium) [long]	2–60	Muscle relaxation, analgesia, anticonvulsant
	Flurazepam (Dalmane) [long]	15–30	Insomnia
Azaperone	Buspirone (BuSpar)	15–60	Anxiety in the elderly; low abuse potential; no sedation

What other pharmacologic treatments are useful?	β-blockers (e.g., 80–160 mg of propranolol), primarily for the autonomic symptoms of anxiety

PROGNOSIS

How long do the symptoms of generalized anxiety disorder commonly last?	In half of cases, symptoms are chronic, and treatment is needed indefinitely. In the remainder of cases, the patient becomes asymptomatic within a few years. A major complication of long-term treatment with benzodiazepines is addiction.

POSTTRAUMATIC STRESS DISORDER (PTSD)

CHARACTERISTICS

Typical patient?	A 50-year-old woman who has survived a car accident in which her husband was killed 2 years previously reports that vivid memories of the event often intrude during her daily activities. She also reports problems in social relationships because she often feels "nervous, distant, and uninvolved."
Etiology?	A catastrophic event affecting the patient or very close relative of the patient that is usually life-threatening or potentially fatal (e.g., war, earthquake, rape, fire, or serious accident)
Symptoms?	Anxiety as well as recurrent nightmares, intrusive memories of the event (flashbacks), increased startle response and hypervigilance, social withdrawal, numbing of affective response, survivor's guilt, and dissociative symptoms
How long do the symptoms last?	Symptoms must last for more than 1 month for the diagnosis of PTSD; in chronic form, symptoms can last for years.
What if the symptoms last for less than 1 month?	Symptoms lasting 2 days to 4 weeks are diagnosed as acute stress disorder rather than PTSD.

DDX

What medical condition is most likely to be mistaken for PTSD?	Head injury caused by the traumatic event
What psychological conditions are associated with PTSD?	Substance abuse, borderline personality disorder, factitious disorder, malingering, generalized anxiety disorder
What is the most salient distinguishing factor between PTSD and these disorders?	Presence of a catastrophic traumatic event in the history
How is PTSD distinguished from adjustment disorder?	The latter is precipitated by a serious (but not usually life threatening) life event (e.g., bankruptcy, divorce).

OCCURRENCE

What is the lifetime prevalence of PTSD?	8% in the general population and up to 50% of people at particular risk, such as combat veterans or rape victims

TREATMENT AND PROGNOSIS

Psychological treatment?	Psychotherapy, support groups, group therapy initiated as soon as possible after the traumatic event. Some success has been reported with EMDR (eye-movement desensitization reprocessing).
Pharmacologic treatment?	There is no good pharmacologic treatment. The following agents have been tried with some success: 1. SSRIs 2. Anticonvulsants, particularly for flashbacks and nightmares 3. β-Blockers, for the autonomic symptoms of anxiety
What happens to patients with PTSD?	Complete recovery occurs within 3 months in 50%; many have symptoms for a year or longer.

Somatoform Disorders, Factitious Disorder, and Malingering

OVERVIEW

What are the somatoform disorders?	A group of mental disorders characterized by physical symptoms without corresponding organic pathology; a patient with a somatoform disorder truly believes that he or she has a physical problem
What are the six major DSM-IV-TR classifications of somatoform disorders?	1. Somatization disorder 2. Conversion disorder 3. Hypochondriasis 4. Body dysmorphic disorder 5. Pain disorder 6. Somatoform disorder not otherwise specified (NOS); persistent physical symptoms (not feigned) do not meet the full criteria for another somatoform disorder. Most common symptoms are fatigue, gastrointestinal complaints, and loss of appetite.
DDx?	The major differential diagnoses of the somatoform disorders involve the possibility that the patient truly has an unidentified underlying physical ailment. Factitious disorder, malingering (in which the patient feigns illness), and psychotic disorders with somatic delusions must also be ruled out.

What three groups of physical illness are most likely to be misdiagnosed as somatoform disorder?

1. CNS illness (e.g., multiple sclerosis, epilepsy, dementia, brain tumor)
2. Early-stage connective tissue disorders (e.g., systemic lupus erythematosus, rheumatoid arthritis)
3. Endocrine and metabolic disorders (e.g., thyroid dysfunction, porphyria, hypoglycemia)

Sex differences in occurrence?

With the exception of hypochondriasis, which is found equally in men and women, the somatoform disorders are more common in women.

Psychiatric comorbidity?

Fifty percent of patients also have another mental disorder; depression and anxiety are most likely to be comorbid.

Etiology?

Genetic influences are found in most somatoform disorders. Although the complaints are not voluntarily produced, primary or secondary gain is often a consequence of the symptoms.

What is the primary gain?

The patient unconsciously expresses an unacceptable emotion as a physical symptom so he does not have to deal with the emotion.

What is the secondary gain?

The symptom allows the patient to get attention from others or to avoid responsibility (e.g., "I am too disabled to drive so you have to drive me").

Can treatment eliminate symptoms?

Treatment can control symptoms, but they often return.

What are the five most useful factors in treatment?

1. Formation of a good doctor-patient relationship by scheduling regular appointments and by reassurance; liaisons with other treating physicians
2. Individual and group psychotherapy, hypnosis, and behavioral relaxation therapy
3. Evaluating the patient's support system and identifying and reducing problems in the patient's life that may aggravate the symptoms

4. Reducing the secondary gain associated with the symptoms
5. Emphasizing management (rather than cure) as the goal of treatment

How useful is pharmacotherapy?

Medications have limited usefulness unless there is a comorbid psychiatric illness, such as depression or anxiety.

SOMATIZATION DISORDER

Typical patient?

A 25-year-old woman has a history of vague physical complaints. She tells you that she has always been ill but that her doctors never seem to identify the problem and are unable to help her.

Characteristics?

Multiple vague physical symptoms lasting more than 6 months including at least
1. 4 pain symptoms (e.g., backache)
2. 2 GI symptoms (e.g., nausea)
3. 1 sexual symptom (e.g., menstrual irregularities)
4. 1 pseudoneurological symptom (e.g., numbness in the extremities)

Occurrence?

Onset before 30 years of age
Specific symptoms vary by culture.

Course and prognosis?

Chronic and lifelong; symptoms are increased by stressful life events

CONVERSION DISORDER

Typical patient?

A 30-year-old woman experiences a sudden paralysis of her legs. She reports the problem in a distant, dispassionate way and notes that her father recently had his leg amputated.

Characteristics?

Abrupt, dramatic loss of motor or sensory function or organ of special sense (e.g., hearing, vision) often with an obvious or symbolic significance

Three most common motor presentations?

1. Paralysis, which shifts to different areas of the body; pathologic reflexes are absent

2. Seizures, which are often bizarre
3. Globus hystericus (i.e., lump in the throat)

Three most common sensory presentations?

1. Paresthesias (abnormal sensations)
2. Anesthesias, which are often inconsistent with anatomic innervation (e.g., "stocking and glove" distribution)
3. Visual problems (e.g., blindness or tunnel vision); evoked potentials are normal (see Chapter 3)

What is "la belle indifference"?

Striking lack of concern despite dramatic neurologic symptoms

Occurrence?

More common in adolescents and young adults, patients from rural areas, and psychiatrically unsophisticated patients

Course and prognosis?

Most patients show symptom remission in less than 1 month, sometimes immediately after hypnosis or drug-assisted (e.g., sodium amobarbital) interview (see Chapter 3); 25% of patients have recurrent episodes, particularly when stressful life events occur

HYPOCHONDRIASIS

Typical patient?

A 50-year-old man reports a history of many "severe and almost fatal" illnesses for which he has visited numerous doctors ("doctor shopping"). When described, the illnesses seem neither severe nor almost fatal but instead represent increased sensitivity to normal physiologic sensations.

Characteristics?

Exaggerated concern with health and illness lasting more than 6 months that persists despite medical evaluation and reassurance

Occurrence?

More common in middle and old age; equal incidence in men and women

Course and prognosis?	Episodic periods of symptoms, each lasting up to a few years, interspersed with periods when few symptoms are present; up to 50% of patients improve over the course of their lives

BODY DYSMORPHIC DISORDER

Typical patient?	A 28-year-old male patient seeks rhinoplasty for his "huge" nose. He avoids social events because he believes others are looking at this abnormality. Physical examination reveals a normal-looking man whose nose clearly fits his facial contours.
Characteristics?	A normal-appearing patient is preoccupied with a defect in appearance, often quite minor. Complaints usually involve slight flaws of the face or head.
Occurrence?	Onset usually in the late teens
Course and prognosis?	Chronic with variable levels of concern over time about the physical feature causing distress Plastic surgery or other medical treatments must be used cautiously because they rarely alleviate symptoms.

PAIN DISORDER

Typical patient?	A 34-year-old woman who sustained a minor back injury 8 months previously, reports serious pain symptoms, although there is no evidence of pathology.
Characteristics?	Patient experiences intense, prolonged discomfort with no physical cause or not explained completely by physical disease; can be acute (lasting less than 6 months) or chronic (lasting more than 6 months); often coexists with a medical condition.
Age of onset?	Usually in the 30s and 40s

Course and prognosis?	Can be disabling particularly if there is a significant physiologic component to the symptoms; patient may become dependent on pain medication. Antidepressants with serotonergic action (e.g., selective serotonin reuptake inhibitors) may be useful.

FACTITIOUS DISORDER (MUNCHAUSEN SYNDROME)

Typical patient?	A 34-year-old man comes to the ER complaining of severe abdominal pain. Examination of his record reveals numerous prior visits to the ER and at least four exploratory abdominal surgical procedures, resulting in a "grid abdomen" due to crossed surgical scars. When informed that no abnormality has been found, the patient dresses quickly and angrily leaves the hospital.
Characteristics?	In contrast to people with somatoform disorders who really believe that they are ill, those with factitious disorder feign mental or physical illness or induce physical illness to gain attention from medical personnel. Patients often have worked in the medical field (e.g., nurses) and have specific knowledge of how to imitate illness effectively.
What are the six most commonly feigned symptoms?	1. Abdominal pain 2. Blood in the urine (by adding blood from a finger stick) 3. Induction of tachycardia (by drug administration) 4. Fever (by heating the thermometer) 5. Skin lesions (by injuring easily reached areas) 6. Seizures
What is factitious disorder by proxy (Munchausen by proxy)?	Simulation or induction of illness in another person, usually in a child by a parent, to gain attention from medical personnel. It is a form of child abuse, which must be reported to child welfare authorities.

Etiology?   Some patients report a history of childhood abuse or neglect, or a serious childhood illness that resulted in medical treatment and/or hospitalization in which the patient felt cared for and protected.

Course and prognosis?   Adult work and social relationships are affected by the preoccupation with illness and medical care; patients may be at risk also from unnecessary medical procedures, medications, and surgery

MALINGERING

Typical patient?   A 55-year-old man who was "rear-ended" in a minor car accident claims that he has "whiplash" and wears a neck collar only when out in public. He reports no further problems after the insurance company pays him a $25,000 settlement but still does not return to work.

Characteristics?   Conscious simulation of physical or mental illness for financial or other obvious gain (e.g., avoiding work or incarceration)

Course and prognosis?   Patient avoids medical treatment and often "recovers" after the gain is realized. Sometimes the disability persists even after a legal settlement.

13   Dissociative Disorders

OVERVIEW

What are they?	Disorders characterized by abrupt but temporary loss of memory or identity or feelings of detachment due to psychological factors
What are the five major DSM-IV-TR classifications?	1. Dissociative amnesia 2. Dissociative fugue 3. Dissociative identity disorder (multiple personality disorder) 4. Depersonalization disorder and derealization 5. Dissociative disorder not otherwise specified (NOS); persistent dissociative symptoms that do not meet the full criteria for another dissociative disorder
Organic DDx?	Head injury, substance abuse, seizure disorder, sequelae of electroconvulsive therapy or anesthesia, delirium, dementia
Psychological DDx?	Posttraumatic stress disorder, malingering
Relationship to cultural factors?	In some cultures or religions, altered states of identity, consciousness, or perception are seen in concert with certain experiences (e.g., trance states entered into at a religious revival meeting); in such contexts, dissociation may not be abnormal.

DISSOCIATIVE AMNESIA (PSYCHOGENIC AMNESIA)

Typical patient?	A 20-year-old woman cannot remember any of the events of a car accident in which she was driving and her sister was killed.

Characteristics?	Inability to remember important information about oneself
Occurrence?	Uncommon; occurring more often in young adults and in women
Etiology?	Use of the defense mechanisms of repression and denial after an emotionally traumatic event
Treatment?	Hypnosis and drug-assisted (sodium amobarbital) interviews (see Chapter 3) to recover the traumatic memories as well as long-term psychotherapy to deal with the recovered material
Course and prognosis?	Amnesia after acute stress may resolve in minutes or days; occasionally lasts for years

DISSOCIATIVE FUGUE

Typical patient?	A 44-year-old man has been living and working in a town 500 miles from his home for over 2 years. He has no memory of his life before this time.
Characteristics?	Sudden inability to remember important information about oneself coupled with leaving home, moving away, and assuming a different identity; the patient is usually not aware that he has assumed a new identity.
Occurrence?	Rare, associated with a history of excessive alcohol use
Etiology?	Traumatic event in the recent past
Treatment?	Hypnosis and drug-assisted interviews
Course and prognosis?	Usually resolves within days, occasionally lasts for years

DISSOCIATIVE IDENTITY DISORDER (MULTIPLE PERSONALITY DISORDER)

Typical patient?	A 32-year-old woman discovers clothes in her closet that she has no memory of

buying and that are quite different from the clothes that she usually wears.

Characteristics?
At least two separate personalities or "alters" (commonly 5–10) within one individual; one alter usually dominates the others

Sex difference?
Most patients are women (although some of the alters may be male)

DDx?
Mild forms may resemble borderline personality disorder or schizophrenia; malingering and alcohol or other substance abuse must be ruled out when the patient presents in a forensic (legal) context

Occurrence?
Not uncommon in mild form; rare in severe form

Etiology?
Early traumatic experiences, particularly abuse in childhood or adolescence; most commonly associated with incest

Treatment?
In some cases, integration of the alters using insight-oriented psychotherapy with or without hypnosis is effective. Antidepressants, antianxiety, antipsychotic, and anticonvulsant agents may be useful.

Course and prognosis?
Often chronic and associated with other psychiatric symptoms, such as depression and anxiety

DEPERSONALIZATION DISORDER

Typical patient?
A 45-year-old woman tells you that she often feels like an observer rather than a participant in her life. She knows that this perception is only a feeling and not reality.

Characteristics?
Recurrent and persistent feeling of detachment from the patient's own body (depersonalization) or social situation, or

from the environment (derealization) with no formal thought disorder

DDx?

Symptoms of depersonalization and derealization are often present in psychiatric disorders such as schizophrenia, depression, anxiety, and histrionic and borderline personality disorders.

Occurrence?

In transient form, occurs normally in many people; there is no sex difference

Etiology?

Severe psychological stress; anxiety and depression are precipitating factors

Treatment?

Antianxiety agents and SSRIs may be useful. Psychotherapy is rarely useful.

Course and prognosis?

Starts most often between 15 and 30 years of age, occurs episodically, and commonly continues for many years

14

Sexual Paraphilias, Gender Identity Disorder, and Homosexuality

PARAPHILIAS

What are the characteristics of paraphilias?

Preferential use of unusual objects of sexual desire or engagement in unusual sexual activity over a period of at least 6 months, causing impairment in occupational or social functioning

Can fantasies be classified as paraphilias?

Only if they are persistent or preferential. Transient fantasies are normal parts of human sexuality. A person who has a paraphilia must have acted on his desires or be preoccupied about them, and must have problems forming close relationships with others because of them.

DDx?

Dementia, schizophrenia, situational difficulties (e.g., lack of suitable available partners)

How common are they, and which are most common?

They are relatively uncommon. Pedophilia, voyeurism, and exhibitionism are most common. Occurrence of some paraphilias is unknown, because they are done privately with consenting partners.

Are paraphilias seen only in men?

Although most paraphilias are almost exclusively seen in men, occasionally pedophilia, sexual sadism, and sexual masochism are seen in women.

Etiology?	Developmental psychological disturbances; possible genetic and hormonal influences
Psychological treatment?	Psychoanalytically oriented psychotherapy, aversive conditioning (e.g., forming an association between mild electric shock and the preferred sexual activity)
Pharmacologic treatment?	Antiandrogens and female sex hormones, so-called "chemical castration," for paraphilias characterized by hypersexuality. SSRIs are also useful.
What two factors predict a better prognosis?	1. The ability to have sexual intercourse in the absence of the paraphilia 2. Presence of guilt about the paraphilia
What two factors predict a worse prognosis?	1. Referral by police rather than self-referral; most paraphilias are against the law and arrests are common 2. Onset at a young age

SPECIFIC PARAPHILIAS

What is exhibitionism?	Exposing the genitals to unsuspecting people in a manner that shocks them
Typical example of exhibitionism?	A 34-year-old man is repeatedly arrested for unzipping his trousers and baring his penis to women on the subway.
What is fetishism?	Sexual preference for inanimate objects, such as women's gloves or rubber sheets
Typical example of fetishism?	A 30-year-old man commonly masturbates while stroking a woman's high-heeled shoe.
What is transvestic fetishism?	Men gaining sexual gratification from wearing women's clothing, particularly lingerie
Typical example of transvestic fetishism?	A 23-year-old man reports that to become aroused, he must wear a woman's nightgown whenever he has sex with his wife.

What is frotteurism?	Men gaining sexual gratification from rubbing the penis against another person who is nonconsenting and not aware
Typical example of frotteurism?	A 28-year-old man is arrested for masturbating by rubbing up against a woman in a crowded subway car.
What is necrophilia?	Sexual satisfaction is obtained from sexual activity with dead bodies.
Typical example of necrophilia?	A 32-year-old man is arrested for murder after he confesses to killing a young woman to have sex with her corpse.
What is pedophilia?	The preferred method of sexual gratification is to engage in sexual activity with children (especially prepubescent children) of the opposite or same sex.
How common is pedophilia?	It is the most common paraphilia.
Is a 15-year-old boy a pedophile if he engages in sexual activity with a 13-year-old girl?	Not according to most state laws, where offender must be at least 16 years of age and 4 or 5 years older than the victim.
Typical example of pedophilia?	A 45-year-old scoutmaster is arrested after an 11-year-old boy scout reveals that the scoutmaster fondled him during a photography session.
What are sexual masochism and sadism?	Obtaining sexual pleasure from receiving (masochism) or causing (sadism) physical suffering or humiliation
Typical example of sexual masochism?	A 46-year-old stockbroker regularly pays a woman ("dominatrix") to beat and humiliate him.
What is telephone scatologia?	Deriving sexual pleasure from calling unsuspecting women and engaging them in sexually explicit conversations
Typical example of telephone scatologia?	A 32-year-old man makes anonymous telephone calls to teenage girls after school hours (but before their parents

return home from work) so that he can talk to them about sex.

What is voyeurism?

Obtaining sexual satisfaction from secretly watching people (often with binoculars) undressing or engaging in sexual activity

Typical example of voyeurism?

A 28-year-old man is repeatedly arrested for using binoculars to spy on women in a neighboring apartment building.

What is zoophilia (bestiality)?

Preferred sexual activity is with animals; can be physically dangerous because sexually aroused animals are often unpredictable

Typical example of zoophilia?

A 25-year-old man prefers to have sexual intercourse with female dogs.

GENDER IDENTITY DISORDER

Typical patient?

A 28-year-old male patient tells you that ever since childhood he has felt like he was "a woman born into the body of a man." He hates his penis and feels like it does not belong to him. He is sexually attracted to heterosexual men, prefers to dress in women's clothes, and would like to have surgical sex reversal to enable him to live his life as a woman.

What is gender identity?

A person's subjective sense of being male or female

At what age does gender identity develop?

Between 2 and 3 years of age

What is gender role?

The expression of one's gender identity in society (e.g., the type of clothing worn in public); may not be concordant with gender identity or biologic sex

What are the characteristics of gender identity disorder?

Commonly called transsexuality, gender identity disorder is a person's subjective feeling that he or she has been born into the body of the wrong gender despite nomal physiology; the person may take sex hormones or seek sex change surgery.

DDx?	Physiological hermaphroditism, schizophrenia, persistent and marked distress about one's sexual orientation (sexual disorder NOS)
Occurrence?	Prevalence is unknown; much more common in men; can be diagnosed in childhood
Etiology?	Unknown; may be associated with abnormal levels of sex hormones during prenatal life
Treatment?	Many patients obtain sex hormones (often illegally) to acquire the desired secondary sex characteristics (e.g., beard, breasts). Supportive psychotherapy is helpful.
How useful is sex change surgery?	Sex change surgery is rarely performed now because depression and other psychological symptoms are often not relieved following surgery, and there is an increased rate of suicide.
Prognosis?	Often, chronic, lifelong distress as well as depression with the risk of suicide

HOMOSEXUALITY

Typical example?	A 45-year-old woman has been living with another woman in a stable, sexual, and loving relationship for 15 years.
What is sexual orientation?	A person's preference for one gender or the other as a sexual and love object
Characteristics?	Homosexuality is sexual preference for people of the same sex
Sexual history?	Most gay and lesbian people have experienced heterosexual sex, and many of them have had children.
Is homosexuality a dysfunction?	No. According to the DSM-IV-TR, homosexuality is a normal variant of sexual expression. Discomfort about one's sexual preference [sexual disorder not

otherwise specified (NOS), which was formerly called ego-dystonic homosexuality] is considered a dysfunction.

Occurrence of homosexuality?

3%–10% of men and 1%–5% of women, but may be underreported; no significant ethnic differences

Etiology?

May be related to alterations in prenatal hormone levels (i.e., increased androgen levels in females and decreased androgen levels in males) resulting in anatomic differences in certain hypothalamic nuclei; sex hormone levels in adulthood are usually normal

Two indicators of a genetic etiology?

1. A higher concordance rate in monozygotic twins than in dizygotic twins and between close relatives
2. Markers on the X chromosome

Treatment for sexual disorder NOS?

Psychological intervention for the person who is uncomfortable about his or her sexual orientation to help the person become comfortable with that orientation; group therapy and specialized support groups may be particularly helpful

Prognosis for sexual disorder NOS?

Homosexual people who are distressed about their sexual orientation (or related social or economic problems) may become chronically depressed

15

Obesity and
Eating Disorders

OBESITY

Typical patient?	A 24-year-old medical student who is 5'8" tall and weighs 260 pounds reports that she has been overweight since childhood. Although she has tried dieting and has lost over 70 pounds on three occasions, she has always gained all of the weight back.
Characteristics?	Being more than 20% over one's ideal weight based on standard height and weight charts
Occurrence?	At least 25% of adults in the United States are obese; more common in women and in people in lower socioeconomic groups
Etiology?	Genetic factors are important; adult weight is closer to that of biologic rather than of adoptive parents
Treatment?	Although commercial dieting–weight loss programs are effective initially, most weight loss is regained within a 5-year period. Gastric stapling, adjustable gastric banding (Lap-Band procedure), and other surgical techniques may be the only effective treatments for morbid obesity (> 100 lbs over ideal weight) even though they have significant morbidity. Maintenance of long-term weight loss is best achieved by a combination of sensible dieting and of exercise tailored to the person's capabilities.

Overeaters Anonymous, a 12-step program based on AA, can be helpful in maintaining weight loss.

Pharmacologic treatments dexfenfluramine (Redux) and fenfluramine (Pondimin) have been taken off the market because their use led to heart valve abnormalities related to increased serotonin levels. Phentermine (Ionamin) is an appetite suppressant that is still used in some patients.

Prognosis?   Associated with increased risk for cardiorespiratory problems, hypertension, diabetes, and orthopedic problems

ANOREXIA NERVOSA

Typical patient?

A 16-year-old girl on the high school track team reports that the school nurse suggested she see a physician because she has stopped menstruating. Although she is 5′6″ tall and weighs 87 pounds, she says that she "should really lose a few pounds."

Name seven behavioral/ psychological characteristics.

1. Despite normal appetite, excessive dieting due to an overwhelming fear of being obese
2. Abnormal behavior in dealing with food (e.g., cutting food into very small pieces, simulating eating
3. Disturbance of body image (i.e., patient feels that she looks fat despite her thinness)
4. Conflicts about sexuality; lack of interest in sex
5. Excessive exercising
6. Abuse of laxatives, diuretics, and enemas
7. Was a "model" child (e.g., obedient, good student)

Name seven physical characteristics.

1. Weight loss (15% or more of normal body weight)
2. Amenorrhea (three or more missed menstrual periods)

3. Metabolic acidosis
4. Hypercholesterolemia
5. Mild anemia and leukopenia
6. Lanugo (downy body hair on the trunk)
7. Melanosis coli (blackened area of the colon due to laxative abuse)

DDx?

Medical condition causing weight loss; major depressive disorder resulting in lack of appetite and weight loss

Occurrence?

0.5% of women; 10 times more common in women than in men; more common during late adolescence, in high academic achievers, in higher socioeconomic groups, and in industrialized societies where there is plenty of food

Etiology?

Societal stereotypes favoring thin women
Interfamily conflicts (e.g., patient's problem draws attention away from parental marital problems)
An attempt to gain control to separate from the mother
Stressful life event (e.g., leaving home for college)

Initial treatment?

Because starvation can result in death, initial treatment is directed at reinstating nutritional condition. If body weight is not too low, this can be done on an outpatient basis using frequent regular office visits and weigh-ins. If body weight falls to 20% or more below normal, the patient may be admitted to the hospital and retained until near-normal body weight is achieved.

Pharmacologic treatment?

Amitriptyline and cyproheptadine [Periactin] (in patients whose body weight is not yet dangerously low); antipsychotics and SSRIs may be effective in some patients

Most effective form of psychotherapy?

Family therapy, addressing in particular the mother–daughter relationship

Prognosis?	Death in 10% of patients from starvation, electrolyte imbalance, or suicide; early age of onset and few or no previous hospitalizations predict a positive outcome; chronically low body weight and obsession with food and eating often continue throughout life

BULIMIA NERVOSA

Typical patient?	A 20-year-old woman comes to see you on the advice of her dentist, who has discovered an excessive number of dental caries. The patient, of normal weight for her height, tells you that when she overeats she forces herself to vomit to avoid gaining weight.

Name seven behavioral/ psychological characteristics.

1. Binge eating (in secret) followed by induced vomiting
2. High carbohydrate intake
3. Abuse of laxatives, diuretics and enemas
4. Excessive exercising
5. Poor self-image
6. Serious concern about gaining weight
7. Distress over the binge eating

Name seven physical characteristics.

1. Relatively normal body weight
2. Esophageal varices (due to repeated vomiting)
3. Enamel erosion resulting in dental caries due to presence of gastric acid in the mouth
4. Swelling or infection of parotid glands
5. Callouses on the dorsal surface of the hand from the teeth because the hand is used to induce gagging
6. Electrolyte disturbances
7. Menstrual irregularities

DDx?	Anorexia nervosa with binge eating and purging (body weight is far below normal); Kleine-Levin syndrome (episodic eating binges and hypersomnia without overconcern about body image or weight gain); borderline personality disorder (poor impulse control including impulsive eating)

Occurrence?	Most common in female adolescents and young adults; 1%–3% of women and 0.1%–0.2% of men; present in up to 50% of patients with anorexia nervosa
Psychological treatment?	Cognitive and behavioral therapies
Pharmacologic treatment?	Average to high doses of antidepressants, including heterocyclics, SSRIs, and monoamine oxidase inhibitors; combinations of cognitive therapy and antidepressants are most effective even in the absence of depressive symptoms
What agents are most useful when there are comorbid mood disorders?	Anticonvulsants and lithium
Prognosis?	At 10-year follow-up, many patients are improved or free of symptoms.

16

Sexual Dysfunctions and Related Subjects

SEXUAL DYSFUNCTIONS: OVERVIEW

Characteristics?	Difficulty with an aspect of the sexual response cycle in the absence of an identifiable biologic basis
What are the four stages of the sexual response cycle?	Excitement, plateau, orgasm, and resolution
Physical characteristics of excitement?	Nipple erection, penile and clitoral erection, vaginal lubrication, and the tenting effect (the uterus rises in the pelvic cavity)
Physical characteristics of plateau?	Increased pulse, blood pressure, and respiration, skin flush on the chest and face, increased testes size, upward movement of the testes, secretion of a few drops of sperm-containing fluid, contraction of the outer third of the vagina, forming the orgasmic platform
Physical characteristics of orgasm?	Further increases in pulse, blood pressure, and respiration, forcible expulsion of seminal fluid, contractions of the uterus, vagina, and anal sphincter (in both sexes)
Physical characteristics of resolution?	Return of the sexual and cardiovascular systems to the prestimulated state over a 10- to 15-minute period
What are the similarities in sexual response between men and women?	Increased pulse, respiration, and blood pressure and appearance of the sex flush during the excitement phase; anal sphincter contractions during orgasm

Which stage is most different between men and women?	Resolution, because restimulation is possible immediately in women but not in men (there is a refractory or resting period in men that varies by physical variables, such as age)
What is the major libido hormone in women?	Testosterone, which is secreted by the adrenal glands throughout adult life
Is estrogen involved in sexual response in women?	Only minimally; menopause (cessation of ovarian estrogen production) and aging therefore do not result in decreased sex drive
How is progesterone involved in sexual response in women?	Contained in many birth control pills, it may inhibit sexual interest and behavior in women
How does stress affect testosterone levels in men?	Reduces levels
How does medical treatment with estrogens, progesterone, or antiandrogens for conditions such as prostate cancer affect sexuality in men?	These hormones may cause reduced sexual interest and behavior through feedback mechanisms.

CLASSIFICATION

What are the sexual desire disorders?	Hypoactive sexual desire and sexual aversion (disorders of the excitement phase)
What are the sexual arousal disorders?	Female sexual arousal disorder and male erectile disorder (disorders of the excitement and plateau phases)
What are the orgasm disorders?	Male orgasmic disorder, female orgasmic disorder, and premature ejaculation (disorders of the orgasm phase)
What are the sexual pain disorders?	Dyspareunia and vaginismus (not due to a general medical condition)

How is presence of a sexual dysfunction determined?	If one or both partners feels that there is a problem
Two major DDx?	1. An unidentified general medical condition (e.g., diabetes can cause erectile dysfunction and pelvic adhesions can cause dyspareunia) 2. Side effects of medication (e.g., SSRIs can cause delayed orgasm), substance use or abuse (e.g., alcohol use can cause erectile dysfunction)
Treatment?	Behaviorally oriented techniques, such as the squeeze technique for premature ejaculation and sensate focus excercises for orgasm disorders Behaviorally oriented psychotherapy, relaxation techniques, and hypnosis (see Chapter 25) Marital counseling and dual sex therapy (both a male and a female therapist see the couple together; see Chapter 26) Medication [e.g., sildenafil citrate (Viagra)]
Who should treat sexual dysfunctions?	Increasingly, primary care physicians are treating patients with sexual problems instead of referring them to sex therapy specialists
When should a physician refer the patient?	When there are serious relationship problems or when there is a history of sexual abuse or rape
Prognosis?	Good, especially if the couple is young and has a pliant attitude

SEXUAL DESIRE DISORDERS

Typical patient?	A 45-year-old woman who has been married for 20 years tells you that she has totally lost interest in having sex with her husband.
Characteristic of hypoactive sexual desire disorder?	Reduced interest in sexual activity
Characteristics of sexual aversion disorder?	Aversion to and avoidance of sexual activity

Occurrence?	At least 20% of adults; more common in women
Three factors in the etiology?	1. Relationship problems 2. Fear of sexual activity due to unconscious factors 3. Normal individual differences in desire
Treatment?	Marital counseling, psychotherapy

SEXUAL AROUSAL DISORDERS

FEMALE SEXUAL AROUSAL DISORDER

Typical patient?	A 26-year-old married woman tells you that although she is interested in having intercourse with her husband (whom she describes as a sensitive and patient lover), she does not become physically aroused when their sexual activity begins.
Characteristics?	Failure to maintain lubrication until the sex act is completed, despite adequate physical stimulation
Occurrence?	Up to 20% of "happily" married women
Three factors in the etiology?	1. Guilt concerning sexuality 2. Anxiety 3. Hormonal fluctuations
Treatment?	Masturbation to prove that sexual excitement and responsiveness are possible; relaxation techniques; normalization of hormone levels

MALE ERECTILE DISORDER

Typical patient?	A 28-year-old man, whose previous sexual functioning has been normal, begins to have difficulty gaining an erection during sexual activity with his girlfriend. Although this problem began after an office party at which he had four alcoholic drinks, he now has the problem even if he does not drink.

Characteristics?

Commonly called impotence, the disorder may be:
Lifelong (i.e., primary: no previous erection sufficient for penetration)
Acquired (i.e., secondary: current failure to maintain erections; normal erections in the past)
Situational (occurs in some situations but not in others)

Occurrence?

10% (lifelong type is rare)
Comprises 50% of total male sexual disorders

Etiology?

Relationship problems
Performance anxiety after previous erectile failure, often because of alcohol use
Increases with age

DDx?

Presence of erections during REM sleep, morning erections, or erections with masturbation suggest a psychological rather than a physical cause

Behavioral treatment?

Lifelong: analytically oriented psychotherapy
Acquired or situational: behaviorally oriented psychotherapy, relaxation techniques, hypnosis

Pharmacologic treatment?

Sildenafil citrate (Viagra), systemic administration of opioid antagonists (e.g., naltrexone) or systemic (e.g., yohimbine) or intracorporeal administration of vasodilators (e.g., papaverine, phentolamine), implantation of a prosthetic device

What is the action of sildenafil citrate?

It increases the availability of cGMP, a vasodilator that helps maintain penile erection when a man is sexually stimulated.

ORGASM DISORDERS

FEMALE ORGASMIC DISORDER

Typical patient?

Although she reports that she is sexually aroused, a 35-year-old woman has never been able to reach orgasm by any means during sexual activity with her husband.

Characteristics?

Lifelong: no previous orgasm
Acquired: present failure to achieve orgasm with adequate genital stimulation (normal orgasms in the past)

DDx?

Incompatible sexual technique, side effect of treatment with an SSRI

Occurrence?

25% of women

Etiology?

Guilt, fear of rejection or loss of control

Treatment?

Sensate-focus exercises in which the person's awareness of touch, sight, smell, and sound stimuli is increased during sexual activity, and pressure to have an orgasm is decreased
Masturbation to identify effective stimulation techniques
Relaxation techniques, including hypnosis
For a lifelong problem, analytically oriented psychotherapy is useful

MALE ORGASMIC DISORDER

Typical patient?

Although he has erections and reports that he is sexually aroused, a 45-year-old man cannot reach orgasm during sexual intercourse with his wife.

Characteristics?

Absence of or retarded ejaculation during coitus despite adequate stimulation

DDx?

Incompatible sexual technique, side effect of treatment with an SSRI

Occurrence?

10% of men

Etiology?

Lifelong: serious psychological problems, guilt due to strict religious upbringing
Acquired: relationship problems, fear of pregnancy or commitment

Treatment?

Lifelong: analytically oriented psychotherapy

Acquired: behaviorally oriented psychotherapy, relaxation techniques, hypnosis, behavioral techniques

PREMATURE EJACULATION

Typical patient?

A 30-year-old man reports that he commonly becomes anxious during sexual activity with his wife and usually has an orgasm and ejaculates just before vaginal penetration is achieved.

Three characteristics?

1. Ejaculation before the man would like it to occur
2. Plateau phase of the sexual response cycle is absent
3. Anxiety is present

Occurrence?

27% of the male population, mostly in young men

Etiology?

May be associated with rushed sexual activity in the past

Behavioral treatment?

The squeeze technique, in which the man is taught to identify the sensation surrounding the moment just before the emission phase when ejaculation can no longer be prevented; at this moment, the man instructs his partner to exert pressure on the coronal ridge of the glans on both sides of the penis until the erection subsides

Pharmacologic treatment?

The SSRIs (e.g., fluoxetine) because they delay orgasm

SEXUAL PAIN DISORDERS

VAGINISMUS

Typical patient?

A 22-year-old married woman has never had sexual intercourse with her husband of 1 year because he is unable to achieve vaginal penetration. Although examination of the external genitalia is

	negative, when you attempt to do a pelvic examination, you cannot readily insert the speculum into the vagina.
Characteristics?	Painful spasm of the outer third of the vagina preventing penile insertion
Etiology?	May be associated with rape or incest in the patient's past
Treatment?	Vaginal dilators in increasing size used in conjunction with relaxation techniques; psychotherapy to deal with the traumatic event in the past

DYSPAREUNIA

Typical patient?	A 28-year-old patient tells you that she experiences severe pelvic discomfort when she and her husband have sexual intercourse. No abnormalities are found during pelvic examination.
Characteristics?	Persistent pain associated with sexual intercourse; may be associated with vaginismus; vulvadynia is a variant
Occurrence?	Much more common in women
Etiology?	May be associated with sexual abuse in childhood
Treatment?	Relaxation techniques; psychotherapy to deal with the traumatic event in the past

SPECIAL SUBJECTS: ILLNESS, INJURY, AND AGING

ILLNESS

How does myocardial infarction (MI) affect sexuality?	Commonly results in erectile dysfunction and decreased libido caused by medications and fear that sexual activity will lead to another heart attack
When can sexual activity be resumed after MI?	In general, when exercise that raises the heart rate to 110–130 beats/minute can be tolerated without severe shortness of

breath or chest pain (i.e., exertion equal to climbing two flights of stairs)

What sexual position is safest for a person who has had an MI?

Those that allow for the least exertion by the patient (e.g., the partner in the superior position)

What is the most common sexual dysfunction in diabetic men?

Erectile dysfunction; orgasm and ejaculation are less likely to be affected.

What are the two major causes of erectile dysfunction in diabetic men?

1. Diabetic neuropathy, which involves microscopic damage to nerve tissue as a result of hyperglycemia
2. Vascular changes due to hyperglycemia that ultimately affect the small blood vessels in the penis

What are the treatments for erectile dysfunction due to physiologic factors?

Sildenafil citrate and similar agents, penile implants, intracorporeal administration of vasoactive drugs, direct application of nitroglycerin ointment to the penis, and systemic administration of opioid antagonists or yohimbine

INJURY

How do spinal cord injuries affect sexual functioning in men?

They cause erectile and orgasmic dysfunction, retrograde ejaculation (into the bladder), reduced testosterone levels, and decreased fertility

How do spinal cord injuries affect sexual functioning in women?

This is not well studied because women receive fewer spinal cord injuries. Vaginal lubrication, pelvic vasocongestion, and incidence of orgasm may be reduced, but fertility does not appear to be affected adversely.

AGING

How does aging affect sexual interest?

Most people continue to have sexual interest throughout life, although availability of partners is often reduced through illness and death

What four ways does aging affect physiologic aspects of sexuality in men?	1. Increased need for more direct genital stimulation to achieve erection and ejaculation 2. Increased time to erection 3. Diminished intensity of ejaculation 4. Longer postejaculatory refractory period
How does aging affect physiologic aspects of sexuality in women?	Vaginal changes, including thinning, shortening of length, and dryness, all of which can be reversed with systemic or topical estrogen replacement therapy

DRUGS AND SEXUALITY

Name three classes of prescription drugs that most commonly negatively affect sexuality.	1. Antihypertensives 2. Antidepressants, particularly the SSRIs 3. Antipsychotics, particularly D_2 receptor blockers
Which neurotransmitter has a depressant effect on sexuality?	Serotonin
Which neurotransmitter has an enhancing effect on sexuality?	Dopamine
Which commonly abused drugs increase sexuality by a disinhibiting effect?	Alcohol and marijuana; chronic alcohol use ultimately decreases both interest and performance
Which drugs of abuse increase sexuality by direct action on the brain?	Amphetamines and cocaine because of their stimulatory effects on dopaminergic systems
Which drugs of abuse decrease sexual interest and performance?	Heroin and methadone

17   Sleep Disorders

NORMAL SLEEP

What does the EEG show in the wakeful state?	Beta (alert, mental concentration) and alpha (relaxed, eyes closed) waves
What are the stages of sleep?	Rapid eye movement (REM) and stages 1, 2, 3, and 4 (non-REM)

STAGES OF SLEEP

What are four characteristics of REM sleep?	1. Dreaming 2. Penile and clitoral erection 3. Increased pulse, respiration, and blood pressure 4. Skeletal muscle paralysis
Most characteristic EEG tracing in REM sleep?	Sawtooth waves
How long is REM latency?	REM latency (time from onset of sleep to first REM period) is about 90 minutes
How long is each REM period?	About 10-40 minutes
How often do REM periods occur?	About every 90 minutes throughout the night
What percent of total sleep time is spent in REM?	25% in young adults
What happens when a person is deprived of REM?	Extra REM ("REM rebound") the next night
What are three characteristics of stage 1 sleep?	1. Lightest stage of sleep 2. Decreased pulse, respiration, and blood pressure 3. Periodic body movements

Most characteristic EEG tracing in stage 1 sleep?	Theta waves (5% of total sleep time in young adults)
What percent of total sleep time is spent in stage 2 sleep?	Largest percentage of total sleep time (45% in young adults) when compared with the other stages
Most characteristic EEG tracings in stage 2 sleep?	Sleep spindles and K complexes
Three sleep-related problems seen in stages 3 and 4 (slow-wave) sleep?	1. Sleep terrors 2. Sleepwalking (somnambulism) 3. Bedwetting (enuresis)
What percent of total sleep time is spent in stages 3 and 4 sleep?	25% in young adults, which decreases with age
Major characteristic of and most characteristic EEG tracing in stages 3 and 4 sleep?	Deepest, most relaxed part of sleep; delta waves

NEUROTRANSMITTERS AND SLEEP

Effects of increased dopamine on sleep?	Decreased total sleep time
Effects of increased norepinephrine on sleep?	Decreased total sleep time and decreased REM
Effects of increased serotonin on sleep?	Increased total sleep time and increased delta sleep
Effects of increased acetylcholine on sleep?	Increased total sleep time and increased REM

SLEEP DISORDERS

INSOMNIA

Typical patient?	A 34-year-old woman tells you that she commonly spends 2 hours every night awake in her bed but cannot fall asleep. The next day she is tired, forgets things, and has difficulty completing her work.

Characteristics?	A problem falling asleep (initial insomnia) or staying asleep (terminal insomnia) that occurs three times per week for at least 1 month and leads to sleepiness during the day or problems fulfilling social or occupational obligations
DDx?	1. Use of stimulant drugs, particularly caffeine 2. Sedative abuser seeking drugs
Occurrence?	About 30% of the general population
Most common etiology?	Medical conditions (e.g., pain and endocrine and metabolic diseases) Withdrawal of sedative drugs (e.g., alcohol, benzodiazepines, phenothiazines, opiates) Use of central nervous system (CNS) stimulants (e.g., caffeine, amphetamines)
Major psychological etiology?	Major depressive disorder
Three characteristics of sleep in major depressive disorder?	1. Normal sleep onset 2. Repeated nighttime awakenings 3. Waking too early in the morning (terminal insomnia)
Four alterations in sleep stages in major depressive disorder?	1. Reduced slow-wave sleep 2. Long first REM period 3. Short REM latency 4. Increased total REM
Characteristics of sleep in mania and hypomania?	Trouble falling asleep and reduced need for sleep
Behavioral treatment of insomnia?	Development of a series of behaviors associated with bedtime, a "sleep ritual" Daily exercise (but not just before sleep) Relaxation techniques Avoidance of caffeine before bedtime Fixed wake-up and bedtime schedule Time-limited use of sleep agents to establish an effective sleep pattern

Pharmacologic treatment of insomnia?	Aimed at the underlying cause (e.g., antidepressants in patients with depression) Limited use of benzodiazepines or other sleep agents to establish an effective sleep pattern (e.g., flurazepam, 15–30 mg) or zolpidem (Ambien, 10 mg) for a 1- to 2-week period
Prognosis?	Depends on the underlying cause

NARCOLEPSY

Typical patient?	A 25-year-old college student falls asleep in class every day and even falls asleep during examinations. She begins to fall asleep as you are interviewing her.
What is narcolepsy?	Sleep attacks in which the patient falls asleep suddenly during the day, despite a normal amount of sleep at night
Three characteristics of narcolepsy?	1. Hypnagogic and hypnopompic hallucinations occurring just as one falls asleep or wakes up, respectively (20%–40% of patients) 2. Cataplexy, in which the person suddenly collapses because of loss of all muscle tone following a strong emotional stimulus (70% of patients) 3. Sleep paralysis, in which the body is paralyzed for a few seconds after waking (30%–50% of patients)
Major change in REM?	Short REM latency
DDx?	Sleep deprivation; sleep apnea leading to daytime sleepiness; abuse of sedative drugs or withdrawal from stimulant drugs
Occurrence?	About 4 of every 10,000 people; most commonly starts in the late teens or early 20's
Etiology?	May have a genetic component

Treatment?	Timed daytime naps Stimulant drugs [e.g., methylphenidate (Ritalin), 10–60 mg/day] (if cataplexy is present, antidepressants may be added); modafinil (Provigil) 200 mg/day
Prognosis?	Danger from automobile or work-related accidents if the patient suddenly falls asleep

BREATHING-RELATED SLEEP DISORDER (SLEEP APNEA)

Typical patient?	An overweight 55-year-old man reports that he is tired all day despite having 8 hours of sleep each night.
Characteristics?	Cessation of breathing for a brief period of time; anoxia, or high CO_2 level, awakens the patient repeatedly during the night resulting in sleepiness during the day; snoring often occurs
What is central sleep apnea?	Litte or no respiratory effort
What is obstructive sleep apnea?	Respiratory effort is present but an airway obstruction prevents air from reaching the lungs; more common than central; a mixture of central and obstructive sleep apnea also occurs
DDx?	Narcolepsy; hypersomnia related to depression; use of sedative drugs or withdrawal from stimulant drugs
Occurrence?	More common in the elderly, obese individuals, and in men
Three most effective treatments?	1. Weight loss (if appropriate) 2. Continuous positive airway pressure (CPAP) 3. Uvulopalatoplasty or tracheostomy (last resort)
Prognosis?	Depression, headaches, and pulmonary hypertension may occur; sleep apnea may result in sudden death during sleep in the elderly and in infants

OTHER SLEEP DISORDERS

What is sleep terror (pavor nocturnus) disorder?	Repetitive experiencing of an extreme form of fright in which a person, usually a child, screams in terror; it occurs during stage 3–4 sleep, and the child cannot be awakened nor remember a dream; commencing in adolescence, it may indicate temporal lobe epilepsy
What is nightmare disorder?	Repetitive, frightening dreams causing nighttime awakenings; it occurs during REM sleep and the person usually can recall the nightmare
What is sleepwalking disorder?	A condition beginning in childhood (usually age 4–8 years) in which the person walks around without being conscious; it is repetitive, occurs during stage 3–4 sleep, and is not remembered
What is circadian rhythm sleep disorder?	Daytime sleepiness due to the inability to sleep at appropriate times
What are nocturnal myoclonus and restless legs syndrome?	Repetitive muscular contractions in the legs and frequent motion of the legs, respectively; both may result in nighttime awakenings; treated with clonazepam (0.5–2 mg before bed)
What is Kleine-Levin syndrome?	Recurrent periods of hypersomnia and hyperphagia, each lasting from 1 to 3 weeks; rare; seen mainly in adolescent males
What is sleep drunkenness?	Repetitive difficulty coming fully awake after sleep even though there has been no sleep deprivation; associated with genetic factors
What is menstrual-associated syndrome?	Hypersomnia and hyperphagia occurring in the premenstrual period

18   Impulse-Control Disorders

KLEPTOMANIA

Typical patient?	A wealthy, middle-aged female celebrity is arrested for shoplifting a video cassette from a store.
Characteristics?	The impulse to take objects without paying for them, despite the fact that they are affordable; the stealing behavior rather than acquiring the actual object is the goal
DDx?	Stealing for actual gain Faking kleptomania (malingering) to avoid prosecution for stealing Conduct disorder in childhood and antisocial personality disorder in adulthood; both have many other behavioral problems Stealing during a manic episode
Occurrence?	Present in less than 5% of shoplifters More common in patients with bulimia nervosa
Etiology?	Family dysfunction in childhood Precipitated by life stress
Treatment?	Aversive conditioning (see Chapter 25) and SSRIs
Prognosis?	Chronic; arrest, legal punishment, and shame are common

INTERMITTENT EXPLOSIVE DISORDER

Typical patient?	A 25-year-old man is arrested for attacking and beating another man while

waiting in line at a store. The store clerk tells the police that the victim had stepped in front of the attacker in the line.

Characteristics? Episodic periods in which the person loses self-control and lashes out without adequate provocation; was formerly called "episodic dyscontrol syndrome"

DDx? Alcohol or drug intoxication
Loss of touch with reality (e.g., psychosis or dementia)
Conduct disorder/antisocial personality disorder
Dissociative disorders
"Amok" is a single episode of explosive behavior seen most commonly in Southeast Asian countries; dissociative symptoms are present

Occurrence? More common in men; familial pattern; onset usually in the late teens or twenties

Etiology? Decreased serotonergic activity, resulting in impulsivity

Treatment? Anticonvulsants (e.g., carbamazepine) and SSRIs (e.g., fluoxetine)

Prognosis? Progresses in severity until middle age; interpersonal and occupational problems are common

PYROMANIA

Typical patient? A 30-year-old volunteer fireman is arrested after it is discovered that he has been setting small fires in vacant lots in his neighborhood.

Characteristics? Repetitive fire setting and overwhelming interest in and attraction to fires

DDx? Insurance gain for losses due to fire
Normal curiosity about fire
Impaired judgment due to another mental condition (e.g., mental retardation)

Occurrence?	More common in men; comorbid with truancy and other antisocial behavior (e.g., conduct disorder) seen in childhood; more common in volunteer firefighters
Etiology?	Family problems in childhood
Treatment?	SSRIs
Prognosis?	Prognosis good for children; poor for adults

PATHOLOGIC GAMBLING

Typical patient?	A 50-year-old man who has made many trips to Atlantic City gambling casinos must sell his house to pay off his gambling debts.
Characteristics?	Pervasive need to gamble that negatively affects family and work relationships
DDx?	Manic episode (obvious mood elevation seen)
Occurrence?	1%–3% of adults; onset at a later age in women than in men
Etiology?	Associated with loss of parent before or during adolescence, childhood ADHD, and major depressive disorder
Treatment?	Gamblers Anonymous (12-step program modeled after Alcoholics Anonymous) is most effective
Prognosis?	Chronic and lifelong; financial problems leading to bankruptcy or theft

TRICHOTILLOMANIA

Typical patient?	A 31-year-old woman must wear a hat in public because she has pulled out all the hair on the left side of her head.
Characteristics?	Need to pull out one's hair, leading to obvious hair loss

DDx?   Alopecia due to a medical condition
                             Obsessive-compulsive disorder, which
                                 commonly is not limited to only one
                                 compulsion

Occurrence?   More common in women; starts in
                             childhood

Etiology   Life stress, depression

Treatment?   SSRIs, antipsychotics (e.g., pimozide)

Prognosis?   Chronic; may last for years; some also
                             show tricophagia (hair eating) leading to
                             bezoars (hair balls), which can cause
                             bowel obstruction.

19

Adjustment Disorders

Typical patient?

When her boyfriend of 2 years tells her that he is in love with another woman and does not want to see her anymore, a 22-year-old woman becomes overwhelmingly sad and cries frequently. For the next 5 months, her feelings of hopelessness are so intense that she misses 25 days of work and often thinks about suicide.

What are the characteristics of adjustment disorders?

Emotional symptoms commencing within 3 months and terminating within 6 months of exposure to a psychosocial stressor (e.g., relationship or business difficulties, retirement, financial setback, physical injury); symptoms lead to impairment in occupational, academic, or social functioning

What are the six subtypes of adjustment disorder?

1. With depressed mood—includes symptoms of depression (e.g., sadness, crying, feelings of hopelessness)
2. With anxiety—includes symptoms of anxiety (e.g., tremor, gastrointestinal symptoms)
3. With mixed anxiety and depressed mood—includes symptoms of both depression and anxiety
4. With disturbance of conduct—includes violations of social norms (e.g., brawling, stealing)
5. With mixed conduct and emotional disturbances—includes conduct disturbances along with depression or anxiety
6. Unspecified—includes maladaptive responses to psychosocial stress such as social withdrawal or work inhibition

DDx?	Acute stress disorder (extremely severe stressor that elicits multiple psychological symptoms, e.g., anxiety, withdrawal, or dissociation lasting up to 2–4 weeks)
	Posttraumatic stress disorder (extremely severe stressor that elicits multiple psychological symptoms lasting more than 4 weeks)
	Normal grief reaction (death of a loved one, which elicits an expected strong response, usually sadness)
	Normal response to stress (psychological discomfort but no significant impairment in functioning)
Occurrence?	Common: 10%–30% of mental health outpatients; more common in disadvantaged populations and the elderly, possibly because of economic stress
Etiology?	Life stress; the severity of the symptoms is not always well correlated with the severity of the stressor
Developmental etiology?	Poor tolerance of frustration and stress because of loss of a parent or poor relationship with parents during early life
Most effective treatment?	Supportive psychotherapy to aid in adapting to the stressful life event and to provide alternative coping strategies
Other treatments?	Group therapy with other victims of the stressor (e.g., other laid-off workers); pharmacotherapy to deal with associated insomnia or depressive or anxiety symptoms
Prognosis?	Depends on the stressor:
	If acute, short latency to onset and brief duration (e.g., no more than 6 months)
	If chronic (e.g., a chronic medical illness), adjustment disorder may continue for a longer period

20

Personality Disorders

OVERVIEW

What are five characteristics of personality disorders (PDs)?

1. Presence of long-standing, rigid, maladaptive pattern of relating to others
2. Presence of personality characteristics that cause social and occupational impairment
3. Lack of insight: individual lacks awareness that he is the cause of his own problems
4. Failure to seek psychological help unless compelled by others
5. Absence of frank psychosis

Do people with PDs have other disabling psychiatric symptoms (e.g., anxiety, depression)?

No, except when the PD leads to difficulties with others.

What are the hallmarks of Cluster A PDs?

The patient is eccentric and/or fears social relationships; includes paranoid, schizoid, and schizotypal PDs

What are the hallmarks of Cluster B PDs?

The patient is emotional, inconsistent, and/or dramatic; includes histrionic, narcissistic, antisocial, and borderline PDs

What are the hallmarks of Cluster C PDs?

The patient is fearful and/or anxious; includes avoidant, obsessive-compulsive, and dependent PDs

Occurrence of PDs?

Each individual PD has a prevalence of about 1% in the population. Schizoid PD may be less common, and dependent, schizotypal, and histrionic PDs may be slightly more common.

At what age do PDs commonly first appear?	For diagnosis of a PD, they must be present by early adulthood. Antisocial PD cannot be diagnosed until 18 years of age (before age 18, it is diagnosed as conduct disorder).
What psychiatric disorders are seen in relatives of PD patients?	Specific PDs are associated with certain psychiatric disorders: Schizotypal (also schizoid and paranoid) PDs—psychotic disorders in relatives Paranoid PD—delusional disorder, persecutory type in relatives Antisocial PD—substance abuse and somatization disorder in relatives Borderline PDs—mood disorders, substance abuse, and antisocial PD in relatives Avoidant PD—anxiety disorders in relatives
Psychological etiology?	Excessive use of maladaptive or inappropriate defense mechanisms (see Chapter 24)
Psychosocial treatment?	Individual and group psychotherapy; self-help groups
Pharmacologic treatment?	No proven usefulness in PDs except perhaps for borderline PD where antipsychotics and antidepressants may be useful; medications can be used to treat associated symptoms such as depression and anxiety Medication must be prescribed cautiously because many PD patients have a high potential for addiction
Prognosis?	Chronic and lifelong

PARANOID PERSONALITY DISORDER

Typical patient?	A 50-year-old office worker tells you that he has never been promoted because his coworkers frequently claim his ideas as their own. When he is fired for poor performance, he files a lawsuit against the company.
Characteristics?	Suspicious, mistrustful, litigious; attributes responsibility for own problems to others

Two major psychodynamic defense mechanisms used?	1. Projection—attributing one's own unconscious, unacceptable impulses to others 2. Denial—screening out of intolerable facts about reality
DDx (and distinguishing feature from paranoid PD)?	Delusional disorder, paranoid schizophrenia, and mood disorder with psychotic features (all include frank psychotic symptoms; see Chapters 8, 9, and 10)

SCHIZOID PERSONALITY DISORDER

Typical patient?	A 48-year-old man is content living alone in an isolated cabin, growing his own food, and rarely having contact with others.
Characteristics?	Lifelong pattern of voluntary social withdrawal
DDx (and distinguishing features from schizoid PD)?	Delusional disorder, schizophrenia (both include frank psychotic symptoms); schizotypal PD Asperger disorder or mild autistic disorder (stereotyped behavior patterns as well as impaired social behavior; see Chapter 5)

SCHIZOTYPAL PERSONALITY DISORDER

Typical patient?	A 35-year-old male patient tells you that he never steps on cracks in the sidewalk to avoid "breaking his mother's back" (magical thinking). He seems odd, says that he often feels uncomfortable in social situations, and has few friends.
Characteristics?	Peculiar appearance, magical thinking, odd thought patterns and behavior without psychosis; many patients are comorbid for major depressive disorder
Two major psychodynamic defense mechanisms used?	1. Projection 2. Denial
DDx (and distinguishing feature from schizotypal PD)?	Delusional disorder, schizophrenia, mood disorder with psychotic features (all include frank psychotic symptoms)

HISTRIONIC PERSONALITY DISORDER

Typical patient?	A 25-year-old female patient comes to your office dressed in a low-cut blouse and very short skirt and brings a gift for you. She fishes for compliments from the office staff and tells you that yesterday she "almost bled to death" when she cut her finger.
Characteristics?	Extroverted, emotional, dramatic, sexually provocative, "life of the party"; inability to maintain intimate relationships; in men, "Don Juan" behavior
Three major psychodynamic defense mechanisms used?	1. Repression—pushing unacceptable feelings into the unconscious 2. Regression—adopting childlike behavioral patterns 3. Somatization (see Chapter 12)
DDx (and distinguishing features from histrionic PD)?	Borderline PD (includes chronic feelings of boredom and emptiness and suicidal behavior) Narcissistic PD (includes feelings of superiority) Dependent PD (not characterized by flamboyance or an overly emotional state) Hypomanic episode in bipolar II or cyclothymic disorder (symptoms remit when the episode ends; see Chapter 10)

NARCISSISTIC PERSONALITY DISORDER

Typical patient?	A 40-year-old male patient tells you that because you are a doctor, you can understand that he is "better than most people." He then asks to be referred to a physician who graduated from an Ivy League school.
Characteristics?	Grandiose, pompous, envious; has sense of special entitlement and lacks empathy

Three major psychodynamic mechanisms used?	1. Denial 2. Displacement—transfer of emotions from an unacceptable to a tolerable person or situation 3. Poor ego functioning
DDx (and distinguishing features from narcissistic PD)?	Histrionic and borderline PDs (include emotionality and instability) Obsessive-compulsive PD (includes feelings of imperfection)

ANTISOCIAL PERSONALITY DISORDER

Typical patient?	A 29-year-old man tells you that he has stolen valuable items from friends and family on many occasions with no intention of returning them and without concern for the people he stole from. He has been unemployed on and off for many years and has been arrested on a variety of minor charges.
Characteristics?	These individuals, who are also known as sociopaths or psychopaths, are unwilling to conform to social norms and fail to learn from experience; associated with conduct disorder in childhood and criminality in adulthood (see Chapter 5)
Major psychodynamic mechanism present?	Inadequate superego functioning (see Chapter 24)
DDx (and distinguishing features from antisocial PD)?	Criminal behavior (includes obvious gain) Substance abuse (may involve stealing to obtain money for drugs) Narcissistic PD (includes needing admiration from others) Paranoid PD (may be characterized by illegal behavior for the purpose of revenge) Hypomanic episode in bipolar II or cyclothymic disorder (symptoms remit when the episode ends)

BORDERLINE PERSONALITY DISORDER

Typical patient?	A 39-year-old female patient tells you on her second visit that she is in love with

you. When you refer her to another physician, she attempts suicide.

Characteristics?	Unstable behavior and mood, boredom, emptiness, feelings of aloneness (i.e., feeling alone in the world, not merely loneliness), impulsiveness, suicide attempts, extreme anger, mini-psychotic episodes (i.e., brief periods of loss of contact with reality); often comorbid with mood disorders and eating disorders

Four major psychodynamic mechanisms used?

1. Denial
2. Displacement
3. Splitting—seeing others variously as all bad or all good
4. Poor ego functioning (see Chapter 24)

DDx (and distinguishing features from borderline PD)?

Histrionic, paranoid, and narcissistic PDs (do not include self-destructive behavior or feelings of aloneness)

AVOIDANT PERSONALITY DISORDER

Typical patient?

A 40-year-old woman who lives alone seems tense and fearful. She tells you that she would like to have friends but is afraid that people will not like her.

Characteristics?

Shy, sensitive to rejection, and socially withdrawn; has inferiority complex

Three major psychodynamic mechanisms used?

1. Avoidance
2. Regression
3. Displacement

DDx (and distinguishing features from avoidant PD)?

Social phobia (experiences significant anxiety symptoms in social situations)
Dependent PD (mainly seeks care from others)
Schizoid PD (is content with little social contact)

OBSESSIVE-COMPULSIVE PERSONALITY DISORDER

Typical patient?

A 30-year-old male patient tells you that his fourth roommate has just moved out because the patient makes unreasonable rules and schedules concerning the care of the apartment.

Characteristics?

Perfectionistic, orderly, stubborn, indecisive, feelings of imperfection

Four major psychodynamic defense mechanisms used?

1. Isolation of affect—emotions associated with stressful events are neither experienced nor expressed
2. Rationalization—seemingly reasonable explanations are given for unacceptable feelings
3. Intellectualization—overuse of the mind to explain away unwanted emotions
4. Undoing—current actions are aimed at reversing past actions

DDx (and distinguishing feature from obsessive-compulsive PD)?

Obsessive-compulsive disorder (an anxiety disorder; presence of actual obsessions and compulsions with anxiety if they are not carried out; see Chapter 11)

DEPENDENT PERSONALITY DISORDER

Typical patient?

A 32-year-old female patient calls your office frequently to ask your advice about obvious, minor medical problems.

Characteristics?

Lacks self-confidence; lets others assume their responsibilities; may be abused by domestic partner

Two major psychodynamic mechanisms used?

1. Regression
2. Avoidance

DDx (and distinguishing features from dependent PD)?

Depression (more episodic and not as chronic); avoidant PD (socially withdrawn)

PASSIVE-AGGRESSIVE (NEGATIVISTIC) PERSONALITY DISORDER

Typical patient?

Two weeks after your 40-year-old male patient agrees that he needs to lose 10 pounds and you spend time describing an appropriate diet, he has gained 2 pounds and tells you that he did not yet "get a chance" to buy the necessary diet foods.

Characteristics?

Stubborn, inefficient; hostile-dependent; procrastinates; seems compliant but is actually defiant (no longer an official DSM-IV-TR diagnosis)

Major psychodynamic defense mechanism used?

Reaction formation—unacceptable feelings are denied and opposite attitudes and behavior adopted

DDx (and distinguishing feature from passive-aggressive PD)?

Oppositional defiant disorder (more directly defiant, usually seen in children)

Subordinate who may not refuse an assignment by a superior

21

Psychosomatic Medicine and Medication-Induced Psychiatric Symptoms

OVERVIEW

What physiologic systems are most commonly affected by psychological factors?

Cardiovascular, gastrointestinal, respiratory, genitourinary, musculoskeletal, endocrine, dermatologic, immunologic, and neurologic systems

In what way is medical illness affected by psychological factors?

By initiation or exacerbation of symptoms

What four psychological factors affect medical conditions?

1. Emotional symptoms (e.g., anxiety, depression)
2. Maladaptive personality styles (e.g., Type A behavior, dependency)
3. Poor health behavior (e.g., smoking, overeating)
4. Chronic or severe stress (e.g., family problems, poverty)

By what three mechanisms do the effects of stress occur?

1. By increasing the release of ACTH, leading to the release of cortisol and depression of the immune system
2. By activating the autonomic nervous system leading to cardiovascular and respiratory changes
3. By altering neurotransmitter (e.g., serotonin, norepinephrine) levels leading to changes in mood and behavior

By which two means can depression of the immune system be assessed?

1. Decreased lymphocyte responses to mitogens
2. Impaired natural killer (NK) cell function

What are the ten most stressful life events?

According to Holmes Social Readjustment Rating Scale, events that require the most social readjustment (including "happy" events) are the most stressful; in descending order:

1. Death of a spouse
2. Divorce
3. Marital separation
4. Incarceration
5. Death of a close family member
6. Serious illness or injury
7. Marriage
8. Losing one's job
9. Reconciliation with one's mate
10. Retirement

What two life events are believed to be even more stressful than death of a spouse?

1. Death of a child
2. Suicide of a spouse

MEDICAL CONDITIONS ASSOCIATED WITH PSYCHOLOGICAL SYMPTOMS

What psychological factor is associated with bronchial asthma?

Excessive dependency

What psychological factors are associated with cancer?

Loss and separation; inability to express feelings

What psychological factors are associated with coronary artery disease and hypertension?

Type A personality, which is characterized mainly by feeling rushed most of the time; competitiveness; and hostility; the latter may be associated particularly with coronary artery disease

What psychological factors are associated with infectious illness and chronic pain?

Depression, stress

What personality type is associated with migraine headache and ulcerative colitis?	Obsessive-compulsive
What defense mechanism is associated with obesity?	Regression, which is the return to developmentally earlier patterns of behavior; e.g., a patient eats sweets whenever he is tense or upset
What psychological factors are associated with tension headache?	Anxiety and depression

PSYCHOLOGICAL SYMPTOMS ASSOCIATED WITH MEDICAL CONDITIONS

What medical conditions are associated with anxiety?	Cardiac arrhythmias and mitral valve prolapse Chronic infections with fever Hyperadrenalism (Cushing's disease) Hyperthyroidism Hypoglycemia or hyperglycemia Pheochromocytoma
What medical conditions are associated with depression?	Pulmonary disease AIDS Brain lesions, particularly in the left frontal lobe Collagen-vascular disease (e.g., systemic lupus erythematosus, SLE) Hypoadrenalism (Addison's disease) Hypothyroidism Hypoparathyroidism and hyperparathyroidism Huntington disease Infectious illness, especially viral (e.g., influenza, mononucleosis) Multiple sclerosis Pancreatic and other gastrointestinal cancers Parkinson disease Vitamin deficiencies
What medical conditions are associated with personality changes?	Brain infections, neoplasms or trauma Dementia Delirium

Huntington disease
Temporal lobe epilepsy
Tertiary syphilis
Wilson disease (explosive anger)

What medical conditions are associated with mania or psychotic symptoms?

AIDS
Acute intermittent porphyria
Cushing disease
Huntington disease
Multiple sclerosis
Neoplasm
Systemic lupus erythematosus (SLE)

MEDICATION-INDUCED PSYCHIATRIC SYMPTOMS

What psychiatric symptoms may be induced by analgesics (e.g., pentazocine, propoxyphene)?

Psychotic symptoms

What psychiatric symptoms may be induced by antidepressants and antipsychotics?

Agitation, confusion, delirium, insomnia, sedation, and sexual dysfunction; precipitation of a manic episode in patient who may have bipolar disorder (antidepressants only)

What psychiatric symptoms may be induced by antianxiety agents?

Sedation, decreased concentration

What psychiatric symptoms may be induced by antiasthmatics (e.g., albuterol, terbutaline, theophylline)?

Confusion, anxiety

What psychiatric symptoms may be induced by antibiotics?

Antitubercular agents (e.g., isoniazid): psychotic symptoms (e.g., paranoia, mania), memory loss
Chloramphenicol and metronidazole: confusion, depression, irritability
Tetracycline: depression
Nitrofurantoin: confusion, headache, sleepiness

What psychiatric symptoms may be induced by anticholinergics (e.g., trihexyphenidyl, benztropine, atropine, scopolamine)?

Drowsiness and agitation
Poor concentration in low doses
Psychotic symptoms in high doses
(atropine toxic psychosis)

What psychiatric symptoms may be induced by anticonvulsants (e.g., phenacemide and phenytoin)?

Mood symptoms, confusion, and less frequently, psychotic symptoms

What psychiatric symptoms may be induced by antihistamines?

Diphenhydramine and hydroxyzine: sleepiness
Phenylephrine and phenylpropanolamine: psychotic symptoms, anxiety

What psychiatric symptoms may be induced by antihypertensives?

Guanethidine, methyldopa, clonidine, and some diuretics: mild depression, fatigue, sexual dysfunction
β-Blockers (e.g., propranolol): depression, fatigue, and less frequently, psychotic symptoms
Reserpine: severe depression, confusion

What psychiatric symptoms may be induced by nonsteroidal anti-inflammatory agents?

Indomethacin: confusion, dizziness, psychotic symptoms, and less frequently, depression
Phenylbutazone: anxiety
Salicylates: euphoria, depression, and in very high doses, confusion

What psychiatric symptoms may be induced by antineoplastics (e.g., fluorouracil)?

Confusion, disorientation, mood changes, depression

What psychiatric symptoms may be induced by insulin and other hypoglycemics?

Anxiety, confusion

What psychiatric symptoms may be induced by antiparkinson agents (e.g., L-dopa)?

Anxiety, psychosis, delirium, mania, depression

What psychiatric symptoms may be induced by cardiac agents?

Antiarrhythmics (e.g., procainamide, quinidine): confusion and occasionally delirium

Cardiac glycosides and digitalis: mild depression and fatigue; delirium is associated with toxicity (particularly in the elderly)

Calcium channel blockers (e.g., nifedipine, verapamil): depression

What psychiatric symptoms may be induced by peptic ulcer drugs (e.g., cimetidine)?

Depression, psychotic symptoms

What psychiatric symptoms may be induced by steroid hormones?

Androgens: aggressiveness, agitation

Progestins: depression, fatigue

Corticosteroids: hypomania and euphoria; withdrawal causes fatigue, depression, confusion, psychotic symptoms; or symptoms such as headache and vomiting imitating a brain tumor—"pseudotumor cerebri"

Thyroid hormones [e.g., triiodothyronine (T_3), thyroxine (T_4)]: anxiety, psychotic symptoms

What psychiatric symptoms may be induced by sympathomimetics (e.g., methylphenidate, dextroamphetamine)?

Anxiety, insomnia, paranoid psychotic symptoms

22

Abuse of Children and Adults

OVERVIEW OF CHILD ABUSE

What are three types of child abuse?

1. Physical abuse ("battered child syndrome")
2. Sexual abuse
3. Emotional neglect (e.g., rejection, withholding of parental love and attention)

How is the incidence of child abuse changing in the United States?

Reported child abuse is increasing, although most cases are still not reported.

What is the physicians' role in these cases?

In all 50 states, the physician who suspects child physical or sexual abuse must report it to the appropriate family social services agency. The physician must also admit the child to the hospital for protection when necessary and arrange for follow-up by social service agencies.

Does a physician have to tell the parents that she suspects child abuse?

No, and she does not need parental consent to hospitalize or treat the child

What are the adult psychological consequences of childhood abuse?

Anxiety, depression, dissociative disorders, posttraumatic stress disorder, substance abuse, and abusing their own children

PHYSICAL ABUSE OF CHILDREN

Characteristics: physical evidence of abuse?

Belt marks, fractures at different stages of healing, spiral fractures caused by twisting the limbs, cigarette burns, burns on the feet or buttocks due to immersion in hot water, bruises on buttocks or lower back (areas not likely to be injured during play), internal abdominal injuries, physical signs of restraint caused by tying to a bed or chair

What is the "shaken baby" syndrome?	To stop an infant from crying, an adult shakes the child back and forth, causing subdural hematomas, retinal hemorrhages, retinal detachment, and sometimes death.
Do abusive parents physically abuse all of their children?	No. Certain children are abused (e.g., those perceived as slow, different, or difficult to control) and others are spared.
Occurrence?	Over 1,000,000 substantiated new cases per year; 2000–4000 abuse-related deaths
Which parent is the most likely abuser?	The mother (who generally spends more time with the child)
Age of the abused child?	33% are younger than 5 years of age 25% are 5–9 years of age
What are four characteristics of the abuser?	1. She was abused as a child or by her spouse 2. She has a substance abuse problem 3. She lives in poverty 4. She and her family are socially isolated
What are four characteristics of the abused child?	1. Child was born prematurely or at a low birth weight 2. Child is hyperactive or mildly physically handicapped 3. Infant is colicky and/or "fussy" 4. Child physically resembles the abuser's absent, rejecting, or abusive spouse

SEXUAL ABUSE OF CHILDREN

Characteristics: specific evidence?	Genital or anal trauma, STD, recurrent urinary tract infection, excessive initiation of sexual activity with friends, precocious knowledge about sexual acts (e.g., fellatio) in a young child

Does the child commonly know the abuser?	Yes. Few abusers are strangers to the child.
Who is most likely to abuse a child sexually?	Vast majority are male; family acquaintance, uncle, father, stepfather, first cousin, older brother
Occurrence?	It is now reported more frequently; 250,000 cases are reported per year
Age of the sexually abused child?	25% are younger than 8 years; highest incidence at 9–12 years
Gender breakdown?	Has been reported in about 25% of all girls and 12% of all boys
What are four characteristics of the sexual abuser?	1. He is a substance abuser 2. He has marital problems and no appropriate sexual partner 3. He is immature and dependent 4. He is a pedophile (occasionally)

ABUSE OF ADULTS

PHYSICAL ABUSE AND NEGLECT OF THE ELDERLY

Occurrence?	About 1,000,000 cases of elder abuse are filed yearly, although most cases are not reported. Not uncommonly, the abused has mild dementia, and/or is incontinent.
Physical evidence of abuse?	Bruises; broken bones, internal abdominal injuries, fractures at different stages of healing, spiral fractures, evidence of restraint caused by tying to a bed or chair
Physical evidence of neglect?	Poor personal care and hygiene (e.g., smelling of urine); lack of needed nutrition, medication, or health aids (e.g., eyeglasses, dentures)
Who is the most likely abuser of the elderly person?	The spouse; if widowed, the daughter or son with whom the elderly person lives and often supports financially
Do elderly people commonly report abuse?	No. Typically, the elderly person says that he "fell" and injured himself.

What is the role of the physician?	To report the case to the appropriate social service agency

ABUSE OF DOMESTIC PARTNERS (e.g., wife abuse)

Occurrence?	At least 2 million cases yearly; many cases are not reported
Physical evidence of abuse?	Bruises (e.g., blackened eyes, bruises on the breasts), broken bones
What are five characteristics of the abuser?	1. He is a substance abuser 2. He has low self-esteem 3. He has a low tolerance for frustration 4. He is impulsive 5. He has displaced his angry feelings about his life onto his domestic partner
What are four characteristics of the abused?	1. She is financially or emotionally dependent on the abuser 2. She has low self-esteem 3. She is pregnant 4. She blames herself for the abuse
What are the three phases in the cycle of abuse?	1. Tension buildup in the abuser 2. Abusive behavior (battering) 3. Apologetic and loving behavior from the abuser toward the victim
What are three reasons why the wife does not leave the abuser?	1. She often has nowhere to go 2. He has threatened to kill her if she leaves; in fact, she has a greatly increased risk of being killed by him if she leaves 3. After the abuse, when the husband is particularly loving, he says he will never do it again and begs her forgiveness; the wife believes and forgives him
What is the role of the physician?	To refer the abused partner to an appropriate shelter or program and encourage her to report the case to law enforcement officials
Is direct reporting of domestic abuse by the physician to law enforcement appropriate?	No, because the victim is a competent adult, and it may put the victim at greater risk.

SEXUAL ABUSE OF ADULTS: RAPE AND RELATED CRIMES

Legal considerations

What is the legal definition of rape?

Rape is known legally as sexual assault or aggravated sexual assault and involves sexual contact without consent. Penetration by a penis, finger, or other object may or may not occur; erection and ejaculation do not have to occur.

Why might semen not be present in the vagina of a rape victim?

Because rapists are more commonly using condoms to avoid DNA identification and HIV infection

Because the rapist may have difficulty with erection or ejaculation

What is sodomy?

Oral or anal penetration (both male and female victims)

Does a woman have to prove that she resisted the rapist for him to be convicted?

No. A rapist was convicted even though the victim begged him to use a condom.

What information about the victim is generally not admissible as evidence in rape trials?

Previous sexual activities or description of "provocative" clothing the victim was wearing at the time of the rape

Can husbands be prosecuted for the rape of their wives?

Yes. It is illegal to force people to engage in sexual activity.

General considerations

What is the typical age of a rapist?

Usually younger than 25 years; the rapist is usually the same race as the victim

How often is alcohol involved in rape cases?

In at least one third of cases

What is the age of the typical rape victim?

Most commonly from 16 to 24 years of age, although they may be middle-aged or elderly

Where does rape most commonly occur?

Inside the victim's home by someone the victim knows

Are most rapes reported?

No. Only 25% of all rapes are reported because of shame or fear of retaliation or problems involved in substantiating rape charges, and blaming the victim is common in rape cases.

How long is the emotional recovery period after rape?

It varies but is commonly at least 1 year; posttraumatic stress disorder sometimes occurs following a rape (see Chapter 11)

What is the role of the physician?

Immediate: Take the history (be supportive and nonjudgmental); perform a general physical examination; conduct laboratory tests (e.g., cultures for STDs from vagina, anus, and pharynx; pregnancy test, test for presence of semen); prescribe prophylactic antibiotics and postcoital contraceptive measures [e.g., mifepristone-RU486 (Mifeprex)]

1–2 Days and 7 days after the incident: See the patient; discuss emotional and physical sequelae (e.g., suicidal thoughts, vaginal bleeding); allow her to talk about her anger; refer her for counseling if necessary; follow up on legal matters

6 Weeks later: Reevaluate her physical status, including repeat tests for STDs (including HIV) and pregnancy; refer for long-term counseling if appropriate

What is the most effective type of counseling?

Group therapy with other rape victims

23 Aging, Death, and Bereavement

AGING

DEMOGRAPHICS

What percent of the United States population will be 65 years of age or older by 2020?

More than 15%

What is the life expectancy of an American?

Overall average is 76 years

What is the gender difference in life expectancy?

Women live about 7 years longer than men. Because men are often some 2 years older when they marry, most married women can expect to be widows for about 9 years.

What is the difference between African Americans and whites in life expectancy?

Whites live longer than African Americans; this difference between the races, about six years in women and eight years in men, is narrowing.

Physical changes of aging?

Impaired vision, hearing, and immune responses; decreased muscle mass and strength; increased fat deposits; osteoporosis; decreased gastrointestinal function; decreased renal and pulmonary function; loss of bladder control; decreased physiologic responsiveness to changes in ambient temperature

Brain changes?

Decreased brain weight; enlarged ventricles and sulci; decreased cerebral blood flow

Are senile plaques and neurofibrillary tangles present in normal aging?	Yes, but to a much lesser extent than in Alzheimer disease
Does IQ change with aging?	No. IQ normally stays the same throughout life. With aging, minor forgetfulness may occur but does not interfere with normal functioning.
How do most elderly people view their lives?	Most have ego integrity (i.e., are satisfied and proud of their accomplishments). Some experience a sense of failure or despair.
Four factors associated with longevity?	1. Genetics 2. Marriage and other social support systems 3. Advanced education 4. Occupational and physical activity

DEPRESSION IN THE ELDERLY

Most common mental problem in the elderly?	Depression; suicide is twice as common in the elderly as in the general population
What three types of losses are associated with depression in the elderly?	1. Loss of family members, and friends 2. Loss of status (e.g., retirement) 3. Loss of health
What condition does depression most closely mimic in the elderly?	Alzheimer disease, because depression in the elderly is often associated with memory loss and cognitive problems (i.e., pseudodementia)
Treatment for depression?	Supportive psychotherapy and antidepressants with minimal anticholinergic activity (e.g., SSRIs and secondary amine tricyclics) and ECT (see below)

OTHER PSYCHIATRIC PROBLEMS IN THE ELDERLY

What are six other common psychiatric disorders in the elderly?	1. Insomnia 2. Adjustment disorders 3. Anxiety disorders 4. Alcohol-related disorders 5. Hypochondriasis 6. Delusional disorder

Why are these disorders common in the elderly?	Because of the losses and stresses of old age as well as anxiety-producing situations, such as physical illness
Treatment of insomnia in the elderly?	Improved sleep hygiene Rapidly eliminated hypnotic benzodiazepines [e.g., temazepam (Restoril)] for short-term use only Nonbenzodiazepine sleep agents [e.g., zolpidem (Ambien)]
Treatment of adjustment disorder in the elderly?	Short-term psychotherapy; drugs are rarely needed
Treatment of anxiety in the elderly?	Supportive psychotherapy antidepressant and antianxiety agents

Treatment of alcoholism in the elderly?	Although often unidentified, alcoholism is present in 10%–15% of the geriatric population. Treatment includes:
	    Supportive psychotherapy
	    Alcoholics Anonymous or other 12-step program
	    Dietary supplements, especially B vitamins, rule out comorbid psychiatric illnesses

Treatment of hypochondriasis in the elderly?	Evaluate the patient for depression; see the patient regularly to investigate objective signs of illness and to provide reassurance
Treatment of delusional disorder in the elderly?	Antipsychotic agents, psychotherapy

DELIRIUM AND DEMENTIA

What are the most common causes of delirium in the elderly?	Physical illness (e.g., MI, cerebral infarction) Vitamin or other nutritional deficiencies Adverse reactions to medications (caused by polypharmacy, decreased metabolic rate and increased sensitivity to medications like anticholinergic agents)
Treatment?	Treat the underlying medical or surgical problem

What psychiatric symptoms are associated with dementia in the elderly?	Loss of cognitive functioning may present with anxiety and depression
Treatment?	Rule out treatable dementia. For Alzheimer dementia, there is no effective long-term pharmacologic treatment, although cholinesterase inhibitors such as donepezil (Aricept) may slow disease progression. Provide a structured environment and treat the associated symptoms (e.g., anxiety and depression) [see Chapter 6].

PSYCHOPHARMACOLOGY AND ECT IN THE ELDERLY

Two most useful tricyclic antidepressants?	1. Desipramine—relatively fewer anticholinergic effects 2. Nortriptyline—less orthostatic hypotension and cardiac effects
Typical dose of these tricyclics in an elderly individual?	Start with a low dose (e.g., 10–25 mg/day), and increase gradually
Why are SSRIs useful?	Because they have fewer life-threatening side effects than tricyclics
Typical dose of SSRIs in an elderly individual?	Start with a low dose (e.g., 10–20 mg/day of fluoxetine or paroxetine; 25–50 mg/day of sertraline) and increase gradually
Two major concerns with using MAOIs in the elderly?	1. Because many elderly are already hypertensive, there are additional concerns if a hypertensive crisis occurs following ingestion of tyramine-containing foods. 2. Drug interactions, particularly with analgesics [e.g., meperidine (Demerol)] and stimulants [e.g., dextroamphetamine (Dexedrine)]
Typical dose of MAOIs in the elderly?	Phenelzine: start with 15 mg/day and increase gradually. Pay careful attention to diet and drug–drug interactions.
What type of antipsychotics are most useful?	High-potency antipsychotics are less sedating; start with 1 mg/day of haloperidol or 2 mg/day of trifluoperazine

Three most useful antianxiety agents?

1. Benzodiazepines (avoid long-acting agents that accumulate in adipose tissue)
2. Buspirone (start with 5 mg/day): less sedation and fewer problems with abuse, but it takes a few weeks for full pharmacotherapeutic effect
3. Antihistamines (e.g., diphenhydramine): provide sedation with fewer abuse problems than benzodiazepines

Is ECT used?

Yes. It is effective and may be safer than antidepressants in the elderly.

How often is ECT given?

A course of eight treatments over 2–3 weeks; afterward maintenance therapy ECT may be useful.

DEATH AND BEREAVEMENT

DEATH

What happens psychologically when a patient discovers that he is dying?

The patient goes through five specific emotional changes, or stages

What are the five stages of dying?

1. Denial—the patient refuses to believe that he has a terminal illness (e.g., "The pathology lab made a mistake").
2. Anger—the patient blames others for the illness (e.g., "Doctor, you should have taken an x-ray last month").
3. Bargaining—the patient uses the defense mechanism of undoing to get rid of the illness (e.g., "I will never smoke again if the tumor goes away").
4. Depression—the patient becomes quiet and sad (e.g., "I feel like giving up right now").
5. Acceptance—the patient comes to terms with his fate (e.g., "I have put my affairs in order and I am ready to go now").

Do the stages always occur in this order?

No. They may occur in any order or simultaneously, or stages may be missed.

Under what conditions other than imminent death will a person go through these stages?

Following loss of a body part (e.g., mastectomy) or with the projected loss of a loved one

NORMAL GRIEF (BEREAVEMENT) VERSUS ABNORMAL GRIEF (DEPRESSION)

What is the difference between normal grief and depression?

After the loss of a loved one or following another major loss (e.g., stillbirth, abortion), there is a normal grief reaction. Normal grieving must be distinguished from a major depressive episode or a dysthymic disorder

How is sleep affected?

Mild sleep disturbances in normal grief
Significant sleep disturbances in depression

Are there guilty feelings?

Mild guilt in normal grief
Feelings of guilt and worthlessness in depression

Perceptual disturbances and thought disorders?

Illusions—most commonly, mistaking a live person for the deceased person—in normal grief
Hallucinations (hearing the dead person's voice) and delusions in depression

Are there feelings of loss?

Expressions of sadness in normal grief
Suicidal ideation or attempts in depression

Is body weight affected?

Minor weight loss in normal grief
Significant (> 5% of normal body weight) weight loss in depression

Does the individual try to return to a normal routine?

Shows attempts to go back to work and social activities in normal grief
Resumes few, if any, social activities in depression

How long do severe symptoms persist after the loss?

Subside within 2 months in normal grief
Continue for > 2 months in depression

How long do moderate symptoms persist after the loss?

Subside within 1 year in normal grief
Persist for > 1 year in depression

**Treatment of a normal
grief reaction?**

Increased calls and visits to the physician,
support groups with other bereaved
people, and supportive psychotherapy
Mild benzodiazepines (but not
barbiturates) for problems with sleep

Treatment of depression?

Psychotherapy, antidepressants, mood
stabilizers, antipsychotics, or ECT

24

Psychoanalysis and Related Therapies

FREUDIAN THEORY

What is the theoretical basis of psychoanalysis and related therapies?

Freud's concept that forces motivating behavior are derived from unconscious mental processes

What are the four types of therapy based on psychoanalysis?

1. Classic psychoanalysis
2. Psychoanalytically oriented psychotherapy
3. Brief dynamic therapy
4. Interpersonal therapy

TOPOGRAPHIC THEORY

According to Freud's topographic theory, what are the three parts of the mind?

The unconscious, preconscious, and conscious

What is in the unconscious mind?

Repressed thoughts and feelings

What is the language of the unconscious?

Primary process thinking

What are the three characteristics of primary process thinking?

1. It is common in young children and psychotic adults.
2. It has no logic or concept of time.
3. It involves primitive drives, wish fulfillment, and pleasure.

What is contained in the preconscious mind?

Memories that are not immediately available but can be retrieved readily and brought to consciousness

Can the conscious mind access both the unconscious and the preconscious mind?

No. It operates in conjunction with the preconscious but cannot access the unconscious directly.

What is the language of the conscious mind?

Secondary process thinking

What are three characteristics of secondary process thinking?

1. It is mature.
2. It is logical and time-oriented.
3. It delays gratification.

STRUCTURAL THEORY

What is Freud's structural theory of the mind?

The mind contains three parts:
  The id (present at birth)
  The ego (begins developing immediately after birth)
  The superego (developed by about 6 years of age)

What is the id?

The part of the mind that contains instinctual sexual and aggressive drives, is controlled by primary process thinking, acts in concert with the pleasure principle, and is not influenced by external reality.

What are the four functions of the ego?

1. To control the expression of instinctual drives, mainly by use of defense mechanisms, in order to adapt to the requirements of the external world
2. To maintain a relationship to the external world
3. To evaluate what is valid (i.e., reality testing) and then adapt to that reality
4. To maintain satisfying interpersonal, or object, relationships

What is the superego?

The part of the mind associated with moral values and conscience

Among the id, ego, and superego, which operates on an unconscious level?

All three; the id operates completely on an unconscious level; the ego and superego also operate on preconscious and conscious levels

What are defense mechanisms?

Unconscious mental techniques that keep conflicts out of awareness, thereby decreasing anxiety and maintaining an individual's sense of safety, equilibrium, and self-esteem

Which part of the mind enacts the defense mechanisms?

The ego

What is the fundamental, most basic defense mechanism?

Repression, in which unacceptable emotions are pushed into the unconscious (e.g., a woman does not remember that she was abused during childhood); all other defense mechanisms are built on repression

What can happen if one defense mechanism is used exclusively or excessively?

Neurotic symptoms can result.

What are "mature" defense mechanisms?

Those that, when used in moderation, help the patient or others directly.

Which four are mature defense mechanisms?

1. Altruism—assisting others to avoid negative personal feelings
2. Humor—joking about negative feelings to avoid the discomfort they cause
3. Sublimation
4. Suppression

Which three are often pathological defense mechanisms?

1. Denial
2. Projection
3. Splitting

SPECIFIC DEFENSE MECHANISMS

What is acting out?

Avoiding unacceptable feelings by engaging in impulsive, attention-getting, often negative behavior (e.g., a depressed teenager burglarizes a store)

What is denial?

Failing to believe facts about reality that are intolerable (e.g., an alcoholic says that he is only a social drinker)

What is displacement?

Transferring emotions from a personally unacceptable situation to one that is personally tolerable (e.g., a man who has unacknowledged anger toward his mother yells at his coworker)

What is dissociation?

Mentally separating part of one's personality or distancing oneself from others (e.g., a woman who was sexually abused in childhood has amnesia for the abuse and five separate personalities as an adult)

What is identification?

Patterning one's behavior after someone else's behavior, either positive or negative (e.g., a woman who was physically abused in childhood abuses her own children)

What is intellectualization?

Using the mind's higher functions to avoid emotion (e.g., as their ship is sinking, the captain explains to his crew the technical details of the damage); associated with obsessive-compulsive personality disorder

What is isolation of affect?

Failing to experience the emotions associated with a stressful event, although the individual can logically understand the significance of the event (e.g., at the funeral, a woman discusses her father's death dispassionately)

What is projection?

Attributing one's own unacceptable feelings to other people (e.g., a man who has unacknowledged and unacceptable homosexual feelings believes other men are lusting for him); associated with paranoid symptoms and ordinary prejudice

What is rationalization?

Explaining one's perception of a negative event in a way that seems reasonable (e.g., a teenage boy who is refused a date says, "I'm glad, we would not have gotten along anyway")

What is reaction formation?

Adopting opposite attitudes to avoid unacceptable emotions (e.g., a woman who is afraid that she will abuse her child constantly buys him gifts)

What is regression?

Returning to behavior patterns characteristic of someone of a younger age (e.g., a man hospitalized for coronary bypass surgery insists that his wife stay overnight with him); seen in patients with dependent personality disorder

What is splitting?

Categorizing people (or even the same person at different times) as either "all good" or "all bad" because of intolerance of ambiguity (e.g., a man who has viewed his doctor as "perfect" begins to hate her when she does not immediately return his phone call); seen in patients with borderline personality disorder

What is sublimation?

Channeling an unacceptable feeling in a personally and socially useful way; a relatively mature defense mechanism (e.g., a woman who is angry at her boss plays a hard game of tennis)

What is suppression?

Deliberately pushing unacceptable emotions out of conscious awareness; a relatively mature defense mechanism (e.g., when asked at a social event about her recent breast cancer surgery, a patient states that she does not want to talk or even think about it—she just wants to have a pleasant evening)

What is undoing?

Believing that one can reverse events caused by "incorrect" behavior by adopting "correct" behavior (e.g., a man who is diagnosed with lung cancer and heart disease stops smoking and starts an exercise program)

PSYCHOANALYSIS

What is the underlying strategy of psychoanalysis?

To slowly uncover experiences repressed in the unconscious mind and then integrate them into the person's personality

What four methods are used in psychoanalysis to recover repressed experiences?

1. Interpreting dreams as representations of conflict between fears and wishes that represent gratification of unconscious instinctual impulses
2. Free association (i.e., the patient lies on a couch facing away from the therapist and says whatever comes to mind), eventually the unconscious is revealed and the therapist interprets the information

3. Analyzing transference reactions (i.e., the patient's reactions to the therapist)
4. Analyzing resistance (i.e., blocking unconscious thoughts from awareness because they are unacceptable to the patient)

What are the six characteristics of an appropriate patient for psychoanalysis?

1. Younger than 40 years of age
2. Intelligent
3. Not psychotic
4. Reasonably stable life situation
5. Good relationships with others (e.g., does not have an antisocial or borderline personality disorder)
6. Able to spend considerable time and money on the treatment

What is the role of the therapist?

To interpret the material produced by the patient during free association

How often is treatment conducted?

Four to five times weekly for 3–4 years

What is transference?

The patient unconsciously reexperiences feelings about important figures in his life in the current relationship with the therapist (e.g., a 40-year-old man who was often disappointed by his mother is extremely angry at his therapist when she is 5 minutes late for an appointment).

What is countertransference?

The therapist unconsciously reexperiences feelings about his own parents or other important figures in the current relationship with the patient (e.g., a therapist who grew up in a poor home feels overly sorry for a patient who loses his job).

RELATED THERAPIES

What is psychoanalytically oriented psychotherapy (including brief dynamic psychotherapy)?

An active form of psychotherapy that is based on psychoanalysis

In what three ways is it similar to psychoanalysis?

1. It is insight oriented (i.e., aims to understand the underlying, unconscious basis for current conflicts and behaviors).

2. It may use dream interpretation.
3. It may use analysis of transference reactions.

In what two ways is it different from psychoanalysis?

1. It is briefer and more direct.
2. Rather than lying on a couch and using free association, the patient sits in a chair and talks directly with the therapist.

What is special about brief dynamic psychotherapy?

Limited to 12–40 weekly sessions, a motivated patient focuses on transference reactions, achieving insight and identifying conflicts relatively quickly.

What are five characteristics of an appropriate patient for psychoanalytically oriented psychotherapy?

1. Motivated to gain insight and understanding, not only to relieve symptoms
2. Able to tolerate emotions that may surface (e.g., anger and guilt)
3. Able to maintain a relationship with a therapist
4. Flexible
5. Intelligent

What is interpersonal therapy?

Based on the notion that psychiatric problems (e.g., depression) are caused by difficulties with interpersonal skills, it focuses on developing these skills in 12–16 weekly sessions.

What is supportive psychotherapy?

Does not seek insight but is designed to make the patient feel protected in an immediate life crisis; in chronically mentally ill patients, it is used for many years in conjunction with medication to provide guidance and emotional support; psychologically well-adjusted patients can also benefit from supportive psychotherapy.

25

Behavioral and Cognitive Therapies

OVERVIEW

What is the underlying strategy of these therapies?	Based on learning theory, these therapies aim to alter behavior and thinking patterns, so that the patient's symptoms are relieved.
How are these therapies different from psychoanalysis and related therapies?	In behavioral/cognitive therapies, the patient's history and unconscious conflicts are not explored because they are considered irrelevant
What are six types of behavioral/cognitive therapy?	1. Systematic desensitization 2. Aversive conditioning 3. Flooding and implosion 4. Token economy 5. Biofeedback 6. Cognitive therapy

SYSTEMATIC DESENSITIZATION

Typical patient?	A 30-year-old woman who is afraid of cats is taught relaxation techniques and is then shown a photograph of a cat. Later in treatment, she is exposed to toy cats, kittens, and finally adult cats.
Most common use?	To treat phobias (irrational fears) [see Chapter 11]
What type of learning is involved in the development of a phobia?	Classical conditioning, in which an innocuous object (e.g., a cat) became associated with a fear response in the past
Purpose of systematic desensitization?	To "unlearn" or counter-condition the association

What is the strategy of this therapy?	Systematically increasing doses of a frightening stimulus are paired with a relaxation response. Because a person cannot be simultaneously fearful and relaxed ("reciprocal inhibition"), the patient shows less anxiety when exposed to the frightening stimulus in the future.

AVERSIVE CONDITIONING

Typical patient?	A 25-year-old man who is a chain smoker is given an electric shock each time he is shown a videotape of people smoking. Later he feels uncomfortable around cigarettes and avoids them.
Most common use?	To treat paraphilias or addictions (e.g., smoking, drinking)
What is the strategy of this therapy?	Classic conditioning. Maladaptive but pleasurable stimulus is paired with an aversive or painful stimulus (e.g., a shock) so that the two become associated. The patient ultimately stops engaging in the behavior because it provokes an unpleasant response.

FLOODING AND IMPLOSION

Flooding: Typical patient?	A woman who is afraid of cats is put into a room containing 20 caged cats and is told to remain there until she is less frightened.
Implosion: Typical patient?	A woman who is afraid of cats is told to imagine being in a room containing 20 caged cats until she is less frightened.
Most common use?	To treat phobias
What is the strategy of these therapies?	Habituation—exposure to an overwhelming dose of the feared object until the person becomes accustomed to it and is no longer afraid

TOKEN ECONOMY

Typical patient?	A 33-year-old mentally retarded woman is given a token each time she combs her

hair. The tokens can be exchanged for goods at the hospital store.

Most common use?

To increase positive behavior in a mentally retarded autistic or severely disorganized person

What is the strategy of this therapy?

Operant conditioning—desirable behavior (e.g., hair combing) increases to garner a reward or positive reinforcement (e.g., the token)

BIOFEEDBACK

Typical patient?

A 34-year-old woman with Raynaud disease is taught to use mental techniques to increase her hand temperature (e.g., imagining her hands in hot water). Her hand temperature is regularly measured and projected to her on a computer screen.

Most common uses?

To treat migraine and tension headaches, hypertension, asthma, Raynaud disease, fecal incontinence, and temporomandibular joint pain

What is the strategy of this therapy?

The patient learns to control measurable physiologic parameters by operant conditioning. Ongoing receipt of physiologic information (e.g., hand temperature measurements) acts as a reinforcing stimulus.

COGNITIVE THERAPY

Typical patient?

A 38-year-old depressed woman is told to replace each self-deprecating thought with a mental image of success and praise.

Most common use?

To treat mild-to-moderate depression, somatoform disorders, eating disorders

What is the strategy of this therapy?

Continuing weekly for up to 25 weeks, a patient's distorted, negative thoughts about herself are replaced with positive, self-assuring thoughts.

26

Group, Family, and Couples Therapy

GROUP THERAPY

Typical patient?	A 45-year-old man whose father was an alcoholic joins a therapy group consisting of children of alcoholics. The group is led by a psychotherapist trained in substance abuse.
What are the three most common types of patients?	1. People with a common problem (e.g., substance abusers, rape victims) 2. People with personality disorders or other interpersonal problems 3. People who have trouble interacting with authority figures (e.g., those who cannot deal with therapists in individual therapy)
How many people are usually in a group?	6–10 is the optimal number
How often do groups usually meet?	Weekly for 1–2 hours
What is the strategy of this therapy?	Members of the group provide feedback, support, friendship, and the opportunity to express feelings.
What is the role of the therapist?	The therapist facilitates and observes the patients' interpersonal interactions, but has relatively little input in the group.
What are leaderless groups?	Peer support groups (e.g., Alcoholics Anonymous, colostomy group, bereavement group)
What is the mechanism of leaderless groups?	Members sharing the same problem provide support, friendship, acceptance, and the opportunity to express feelings

FAMILY THERAPY

Typical patient?

A 16-year-old girl with anorexia nervosa, her parents, and her two siblings meet with a therapist weekly for a 2-hour session.

What are the four most common problems treated with this therapy?

1. Eating disorders
2. Behavioral problems in children
3. Substance abuse
4. Family conflicts

What is the strategy of this therapy?

Addressing the notion that psychopathology in one family member (i.e., the identified patient) reflects dysfunction of the entire family system. Because circular rather than linear causality results in symptoms, the family (rather than the individual with the problem) is really the patient.

What three family characteristics are identified in family therapy?

1. Dyads: subsystems between two family members, such as the "executive subsystem" containing the two parents
2. Triangles: dysfunctional alliances between two family members against a third member, such as a coalition of father and daughter against mother
3. Boundaries: obstruction between subsystems, such as the barrier between the executive subsystem and the children; may be too rigid or too permeable

What three processes are encouraged in family therapy?

1. Mutual accommodation, a process in which family members learn each other's needs and work toward meeting those needs
2. Redefining "blame" and encouraging family members to reconsider their own responsibility for problems, thereby relieving symptoms in the identified patient
3. Normalizing boundaries between subsystems

COUPLES THERAPY

Typical patients?	A husband and wife who have been married for 15 years have not had sex in 10 months, argue constantly, and are contemplating divorce.
What are the three most common reasons for couples therapy?	1. Communication problems 2. Psychosexual problems 3. Differences in values
What are the four types?	1. Conjoint therapy: one therapist sees the couple together (most common type) 2. Concurrent therapy: one therapist sees both members of the couple individually 3. Collaborative therapy: two therapists (usually one for each member of the couple) see both members of the couple individually 4. Four-way therapy: two therapists (one for each member of the couple) see the couple together; used most commonly for sexual problems

27

Psychiatric Problems in Medical Patients: Consultation–Liaison Psychiatry

OVERVIEW

Typical patient?

A woman who has an active genital herpes infection is in labor. She tells her obstetrician that she will not consent to a cesarean section delivery, because her mother died during a surgical procedure.

What are the nine most common problems treated by consultation-liaison (CL) psychiatrists?

1. Noncompliance with medical advice or treatment
2. Refusal to consent to needed medical or surgical procedures
3. Depression and suicidal threats
4. Anxiety
5. Sleep disorders
6. Disorientation (often the result of delirium)
7. Chronic psychiatric illness in a medical patient
8. Medical complications of psychotropic agents
9. Medical complications of a suicide attempt

Which five groups of hospitalized patients are at highest risk for psychological problems?

1. ICU patients
2. Postoperative patients
3. Renal dialysis patients
4. Surgical patients
5. AIDS patients

What are three types of psychosocial intervention provided by CL psychiatrists?	1. Short-term, dynamic psychotherapy (see Chapter 26) to deal with the immediate problem 2. Identifying and organizing the patient's social support systems 3. Developing methods of dealing with real social/occupational problems

ICU PATIENTS

What is the major risk of psychological problems?	Because these patients are seriously ill, their clinical stability may be threatened by psychological problems.
What problems are ICU patients most at risk for?	Delirium (ICU psychosis) and depression
What are two ways to reduce psychological and medical risk?	1. Enhance sensory input (e.g., good lighting, provide photos of family members) 2. Allow the patient to manage her environment (e.g., control over lighting, pain medication) as much as possible

AIDS PATIENTS

What are four reasons for psychological problems in AIDS patients?	1. The illness is potentially fatal. 2. Guilt that they may have engaged in behavior that led to the illness (e.g., IV drug abuse) and may have given the virus to others 3. The need to "come out" (i.e., reveal their sexual orientation) to others if they are homosexual 4. The need to deal with others' fears of contagion
How can psychological and medical risk be reduced?	Provide access to psychological counseling

RENAL DIALYSIS PATIENTS

Why are they at risk for psychological problems?	Because they must depend on machines and other people

What are the three most common problems?

Depression, suicide, and sexual dysfunction

How can psychological and medical risk be reduced?

Use of in-home rather than in-hospital dialysis units, reducing disruption of the patient's lifestyle

SURGICAL PATIENTS

Which three groups of surgical patients are at highest risk for morbidity and mortality?

1. Those who believe that they will not survive surgery
2. Those who deny that they are worried before surgery
3. Those who have unrealistic expectations of surgery

What are four ways to reduce psychological and medical risk?

1. Develop a positive attitude in the patient toward the surgery
2. Allow and encourage the patient to talk about her fears and depression
3. Explain what the patient can expect during and after the procedure (e.g., mechanical support, pain)
4. Explain and ensure that the patient understands the likely outcome of the surgery

28

Medicine and Law

MEDICAL MALPRACTICE

Typical patient?

A 35-year-old man receives a spinal anesthetic for knee surgery. Following the surgery, the patient has partial paralysis of the affected leg and sues the anesthesiologist for malpractice.

Will the lawsuit be successful?

Yes, if the patient can prove that the physician committed the four "Ds" of malpractice. An unfavorable outcome alone (e.g., the paralysis) does not constitute malpractice.

What is medical malpractice?

A physician causes harm to a patient by deviating from an accepted standard of practice

Is malpractice a crime?

No. Malpractice is a tort, or civil wrong, not a crime.

What are the "four Ds" of malpractice?

Dereliction (negligence; e.g., deviation from normal standards of professional care) of a

Duty (there was an established doctor–patient relationship) causing

Damages (the patient was injured in some way)

Directly to the patient (also known as "proximate cause," meaning that the damages were caused by the negligence, not by another factor)

What are compensatory damages?

Money awarded to the patient to reimburse him for:

Medical bills and lost salary (economic damages)

Pain and suffering (noneconomic damages)

What are punitive (or exemplary) damages?	Money awarded to the patient for the purpose of punishing the doctor and setting an example for the medical community. Punitive damages are rare and awarded only in cases of wanton carelessness or gross negligence (e.g., a drunk surgeon cuts a vital nerve).
Which two medical specialists are most likely to be sued for malpractice?	Surgical specialists (including obstetricians) and anesthesiologists
Which two medical specialists are least likely to be sued?	Psychiatrists and family practitioners
Are sexual relationships with patients or former patients ever appropriate?	No. Sexual relations with current or former patients are considered inappropriate acts that are a form of malpractice proscribed by the published ethical standards of most specialty boards. There may be a time limit on the definition of former patient.
How do patients pursue sexual complaints?	Patients who claim a sexual relationship may file an ethics complaint against the doctor and/or file a medical malpractice complaint.
How do malpractice insurance carriers usually respond?	Many will not pay a judgment based on improper sexual behavior even if they agree to pay for a legal defense.
What are three reasons for the increase in malpractice claims?	1. General increase in lawsuits 2. Heightened expectations that patients have of doctors 3. Breakdown of the traditional physician–patient relationship because of the increased technological base of medicine, less time for personal interaction, and limited physician autonomy because of managed care

ADVANCE DIRECTIVES

Typical patient?	A 75-year-old woman signs a document (a living will) stating that if she enters a persistent vegetative state, she does not

want heroic measures taken to save her life. Two weeks later, she goes into a coma. Her daughter urges the physician to save her mother's life.

Should the doctor take heroic measures?

Not unless he expects her to recover; the daughter's wishes are not relevant to his decision

What are the two major types of advance directives?

1. Living will
2. Durable power of attorney

What is a living will?

A document in which a patient gives directions for future health care if she is incompetent to make decisions at the time care is required

What is a durable power of attorney?

A document in which a patient designates another person (e.g., her husband) as her legal representative to make decisions concerning her health care when she can no longer do so

What are two requirements of hospitals and nursing homes with respect to advance directives?

1. They must inform patients of their right to refuse treatment or resuscitation
2. They must inquire about and assist patients in writing advance directives

Which hospitals and nursing homes have these two requirements?

Those receiving Medicare payments (most institutions do)

What standard is used for incompetent patients who have no advance directives?

Health care providers or family members (surrogates) must determine what the patient would have done if she were competent (the substituted judgment standard) or what a reasonable person would do after weighing each course of action (the best interest standard).

What about the personal wishes of surrogates?

They are not relevant to the medical decision.

DEFINITION OF DEATH

Typical patient?

A 35-year-old woman sustains head injuries in an automobile accident. She is in a coma on a life-support system. Her husband asks the physician not to turn off the life-support machines.

Should this woman be maintained on a life-support system?

If there is irreversible cessation of brain function, this patient is legally dead and life support can be turned off. Provide support and counseling to the husband to help him accept the death.

What is a physician's role when a person dies?

To certify the cause of death (e.g., natural, suicide, accident)
To sign the death certificate

What is the legal definition of death in the United States?

Irreversible cessation of all functions of the entire brain, including the brain stem

May food, water, medical care, and artificial life support be withheld from a patient who has no realistic chance of regaining consciousness but is not legally dead?

Yes. Under appropriate circumstances, indirect or "passive" euthanasia is an acceptable procedure for a comatose terminally ill patient with no reasonable prospect of recovery.

Is it legal or ethical, neither legal nor ethical, or both legal and ethical for a physician to halt artificial life support systems if requested to do so by a competent patient?

Both legal and ethical

According to medical codes of ethics (American Medical Association, medical specialty organizations), is active euthanasia an acceptable procedure?

Active euthanasia is a criminal act that is never appropriate.

INVOLUNTARY HOSPITALIZATION OF PSYCHIATRIC PATIENTS

Typical patient?

A 35-year-old paranoid schizophrenic woman, who lives in a cardboard box under a bridge, is brought to the emergency room dirty, disheveled, and malnourished. She refuses to be hospitalized.

Can this woman be involuntarily hospitalized?

Not unless she poses a significant danger to herself or others; self-neglect is not grounds for involuntary hospitalization unless it constitutes a significant, imminent danger to her life

What are two types of admission to a mental health facility?

1. Voluntary: used for patients who choose to be hospitalized; however, unlike most medical admissions, voluntary psychiatric patients must wait 24–48 hours before they are permitted to sign out against advice
2. Emergency or involuntary: used for patients who will not or cannot agree to be hospitalized; requires the certification of one physician (emergency hospitalization: "one physician certificate") or two physicians ("two physician certificate")

How long can the patient be held in an involuntary admission before a court hearing?

15 days for emergency hospitalization, 60 days for involuntary hospitalization depending on state laws. The court may repeatedly extend the confinement for 3 months or more at a time.

What are seven rights of patients confined to mental health facilities (Mental Health Bill of Rights)?

1. Right to receive appropriate treatment
2. Right to refuse treatment (e.g., medication, electroconvulsive therapy, surgical procedures) unless it is determined to be necessary to prevent danger to the patient or to others
3. Right to privacy
4. Right to manage one's own finances, unless declared legally incompetent
5. Right to receive visitors
6. Right to communicate with the outside world
7. Right to be paid for work done in the facility

CRIMINAL LAW

Typical patient?

A 29-year-old schizophrenic man is arrested for murdering a 9-year-old boy.

The man says that God told him to kill the boy because the boy was "the Devil" (a "command" hallucination).

Did the man commit a crime?

Although this man committed an illegal act (i.e., homicide), the act alone is not necessarily a crime. To constitute a crime, there must be evil intent (*mens rea*) as well as an evil deed (*actus reus*). In this case, a judge or jury may determine that the man lacked the requisite state of mind to have committed a crime.

Who is competent to stand trial?

Everyone is presumed competent unless he does not understand the charges against him or is not able to cooperate with counsel in the preparation of his defense.

What are two major requirements for a person to be found legally insane?

1. He has a mental illness, AND
2. As a consequence of the mental illness, he meets one of the statutory criteria under state or federal law

What is diminished capacity?

A qualification in some states or federal jurisdictions under which a mentally ill person is charged with a reduced level of crime or has his punishment modified

STATUTORY CRITERIA FOR LEGAL INSANITY AS A RESULT OF MENTAL ILLNESS

What is the *M'Naghten* test?

Does the person understand the nature and quality of his actions? If so, does he know the actions were wrong? This is the strictest test, and it is the standard criterion in most jurisdictions.

What is the American Law Institute (ALI) Model Penal Code test?

Does the person appreciate the wrongfulness of his behavior (cognitive prong)? Alternatively, is he able to conform his conduct to the requirements of the law (volitional prong; after the John Hinckley case, most jurisdictions dropped this alternative.)

What is the *Durham* test?

Is the person's criminal behavior the "product" of a mental illness? This is the

most lenient test, and it has been
abandoned in almost all jurisdictions.

THE RIGHT TO DIE AND RELATED ISSUES

Typical patient?

A 28-year-old woman and her 7-year-old
child are in a serious automobile accident.
Both of them need blood transfusions.
The woman, who is lucid, tells you that it
is against her religion to receive blood
and that she refuses the transfusions for
both herself and the child.

**Does the physician have to
abide by the woman's
wishes?**

Assuming the woman is competent, she
can refuse lifesaving treatment for herself
based on religious or other reasons, even
if death will be the outcome. However,
the mother (or the father) cannot refuse
lifesaving treatment for the minor child
for any reason; if it is not an emergency
situation, a court order to treat the child
must be obtained. In an emergency, the
physician can proceed without a court
order.

**What is the legal definition
of competence for
accepting or refusing
medical treatment?**

The patient understands the risks and
benefits of the medical treatment offered
and what is likely to happen if the
treatment is refused.

**Can a person be mentally
ill or retarded and
competent to agree to
medical treatment?**

Yes, as long as he meets the legal
standard, even if he is incompetent in
other areas of life (e.g., with finances)

**Can a competent woman
refuse treatment (e.g.,
cesarean section) aimed at
saving the life of her fetus?**

Yes, even if death or serious injury to the
fetus will result

**Is physician-assisted
patient suicide (e.g., Dr.
Kevorkian cases) legal?**

Although not "strictly legal" in any state,
it is not generally an indictable offense as
long as the physician does not carry out
the killing herself (i.e., active euthanasia).

29

Medical Ethics

INFORMED CONSENT

INFORMED CONSENT IN THE TREATMENT OF ADULTS

Typical patient?	You discover that an 80-year-old man with a heart condition has prostate cancer that requires treatment. His wife tells you not to tell him the truth about his diagnosis because "if it is cancer, it will kill him."
Should you tell him the diagnosis?	Yes. Ordinarily you must provide a patient with full information about his diagnosis in order to obtain informed consent for his treatment. However, if in your medical opinion you believe that his life or health will be at risk if you tell him, you do not have to do so until the potential for adverse effects is reduced. The opinions of family members are not considered legally relevant, however.
Who obtains consent?	The physician (other hospital personnel such as nurses generally cannot obtain informed consent), before any medical or surgical procedure
What four things must the patient understand before he can give informed consent?	1. The diagnosis or the medical finding 2. The treatment, alternatives to treatment, and risks and benefits of treatment 3. What is likely to happen if he does not consent to the procedure 4. That he can withdraw consent at any time before the procedure (even on the way to the operating room after preanesthetic medication has been given)

Is a signed document required?	Although a signature is not necessarily required for minor medical procedures, the patient should be required to sign a document of agreement for major medical procedures or for surgery.
What if there is an unexpected finding during surgery requiring a non-emergency procedure the patient has not consented to (e.g., an unexpected positive breast biopsy requiring mastectomy)?	The patient must be allowed to wake up and give a new informed consent before the additional procedure can be performed.
What if there is an unexpected finding requiring an emergency procedure (e.g., an unexpected "hot" appendix found during surgery for an ovarian cyst)?	The surgeon should do the emergency procedure without informed consent.

INFORMED CONSENT IN THE TREATMENT OF MINORS

At what age is an individual usually no longer a minor?	18 years of age, unless emancipated (see below)
Typical patient?	A 15 year-old-girl breaks her arm while playing basketball in the school gym.
Can the teacher or school principal give consent for the girl's medical treatment?	No. Only the parent or legal guardian can give consent for medical treatment of a minor.
What if the parent or guardian cannot be located?	Medical treatment may proceed without consent, but only to the extent that the treatment is considered an emergency. Some schools ask parents to sign a blanket consent form at the start of the school year, but these forms have questionable legal validity.
Can you treat chlamydia in a 15-year-old without obtaining consent from her parents?	Yes. Most state laws create an exception in which you can treat a minor for an STD without telling the parent and without obtaining parental consent.

Under what four other circumstances is parental consent not required?	1. In emergency situations 2. For providing medical care during pregnancy 3. For providing contraceptives 4. For treating drug and alcohol dependence
Is parental consent required when a minor seeks an abortion?	Most states require the notification or consent of one or both parents.
What if parents refuse to consent to established medical treatment for religious or other reasons when their child's life is threatened by a medical illness or accident?	A parent or guardian cannot refuse needed, lifesaving treatment for a child.
What must you do to treat the child when the parents refuse consent?	Obtain a court order if there is time to do so (i.e., at least a few hours); if not, proceed with the treatment.
Will courts order experimental or nonestablished procedures for children?	No
Under what three conditions are minors considered emancipated and can give their own consent for their own medical care?	1. If they are married 2. If they are self-supporting or in the military 3. If they have children whom they care for

CONFIDENTIALITY

Typical patient?	A patient tells you that as soon as he gets out of the hospital, he is going to kill himself. He begs you not to tell anyone.
Are you ethically required to keep this information confidential?	Although doctors are expected to maintain patient confidentiality, they do not have to do so if the patient is at significant risk for suicide.

Under what two other circumstances can you break physician–patient confidentiality?	1. When the patient is suspected of child or elder abuse 2. When the patient poses a serious risk to another person (e.g., an angry patient is threatening a neighbor)
What do you do if a patient makes a serious threat toward another person?	Determine the credibility of the threat. If credible, the physician must take appropriate action, such as warning the intended victims, notifying law enforcement officials or social service agencies or arranging for committing the patient (the *Tarasoff* decision).

REPORTABLE ILLNESSES

Typical patient?	You discover that your 34-year-old female patient has genital herpes. Her boyfriend asks you what is wrong with her.
Do you have to tell him the diagnosis?	You do not have to tell sexual partners unless their health or life is in danger because of the patient's behavior. You should, however, encourage the patient to tell the partner.
Do you have to report the case? If so, to whom?	No. Genital herpes generally does not have to be reported to state health authorities.
What illnesses are reportable to state health authorities?	It differs state by state, but in most states reportable conditions include AIDS (but not HIV-positive status) and some STDs, such as syphilis and gonorrhea; like genital herpes, chlamydia is generally not reportable. Reportable diseases also include hepatitis A and B, salmonellosis, shigellosis, tuberculosis, chicken pox, measles, mumps, and rubella.
Does the physician report such illnesses directly to the federal Centers for Disease Control and Prevention (CDC)?	No. The physician must report only to the state department of health. For statistical purposes, states report these illnesses without patient names to the CDC.

ETHICAL ISSUES IN HIV INFECTION

Typical scenario?	A 34-year-old female physician refuses to treat a 25-year-old male HIV-positive patient because he poses a risk to her.
Is her refusal ethical?	No. She may not refuse to treat him for this reason.
Must a physician knowingly exposed to HIV be tested?	Medically and ethically, yes, but not legally.
Can an HIV-positive doctor treat patients?	Yes, provided he is physically and mentally competent to do so and that he complies with precautions for infection control.
Does an HIV-positive doctor have to reveal his positive status to his patients and to the medical community?	No
What should a physician do when an HIV+ patient reveals that he is having unprotected sex?	Encourage the patient to disclose his HIV+ status to his sexual partner and set up an appointment for both in the physician's office to be sure he follows through and to answer the partner's questions.
What if the patient refuses to tell his partner?	The doctor must tell the partner because the patient's behavior poses a significant risk to the partner's life.

IMPAIRED PHYSICIANS

Typical scenario?	On your surgical rotation, you frequently smell alcohol on the breath of another medical student. You talk to her but she denies having a problem with alcohol.
What should you do?	Report her to the dean of students or the dean of the medical school or confer with the state medical committee for impaired physicians. In the case of an impaired resident or attending physician, report to the director of residency training or the chief of the medical staff, respectively.

What are the most common causes of impairment in physicians?

Drug or alcohol abuse, boundary violations, physical illness, mental illness, impairment in functioning due to old age

Is reporting of an impaired colleague required legally?

It varies by state.

Is reporting of an impaired colleague required ethically?

Yes. Patients must be protected and the impaired colleague must be helped.

To whom do you report the colleague if you are both licensed physicians?

The state licensing board or the impaired physicians' program, usually part of the state medical society

Glossary of Psychiatric Terms and Abbreviations

Abulia	Lack of volition
Acting out	Impulsive, often dramatic behavior as a result of unconscious mental processes
Affect	External (facial) reflection of internal feelings
Agitation	Physical restlessness often as a result of emotional discomfort; can be a side effect of medication
Agnosia	Problems in recognition of sensory stimuli (e.g., in visual agnosia a patient cannot identify familiar people or familiar objects)
Agoraphobia	Fear of open, unprotected places or of places where escape is unlikely
Agranulocytosis	Decreased number of white blood cells, particularly polymorphonuclear leukocytes
Agraphia	Inability to write or deficits in construction of words
Akathisia	Subjective feeling of motor restlessness
Akinesia	Absence of movement often due to psychological causes; can be a side effect of medication
Alexia	Inability to read despite normal vision
Ambivalence	Feeling two different and opposite ways about the same situation at the same time
Amnesia	Difficulty recalling important personal information
Amotivational syndrome	Lack of drive to advance in life, often attributable to use of drugs of abuse (e.g., marijuana)
Anaclitic depression	Apathy, poor growth, and social withdrawal in a child due to failure of normal parent–child bonding; also called "failure to thrive" and reactive attachment disorder

Anhedonia	Complete absence of the ability to feel pleasure; seen in severe depressive states
Anomia	Inability to name objects
Anterograde amnesia	Inability to learn new material or to encode new information in memory
Anxiety	Symptoms of fear without logical cause
Aphasia	Difficulty with verbal comprehension (receptive) or verbal expression (expressive)
Apathy	Lack of interest in others or the environment
Apperception	Alteration of perceptual experiences by emotions
Apraxia	Problems following instructions to complete tasks; not due to mental retardation or physical disability
Ataxia	Abnormal muscular coordination
Auditory hallucination	Subjective perception of sound without auditory stimulus; commonly seen in schizophrenia
Autism	Complete self-involvement in a private world
Automatism	Carrying out stereotyped acts in a robot-like, automatic fashion
Bereavement (grief)	Sadness due to an actual loss
Blocking	Sudden halt in the train of thought
Blunted affect	Strongly decreased display of emotions
Bradykinesia	Slowed movements
Broca's aphasia	Problems with verbal expression due to a dominant frontal lobe lesion
Catalepsy	State of complete immobility
Cataplexy	Sudden loss of all motor control; seen in narcolepsy
Catatonia	Motor problems such as rigidity, posturing, or excitement due to psychological causes
Cenesthesic (somatic) hallucination	Hallucination that something (e.g., burning or cutting) is taking place inside the body

Circumstantiality	Tendency to include too many details and irrelevant facts in speech
Clang association	Repeated use of rhyming words or phrases
Clouding of consciousness	Loss of ability to respond normally to external events, as in delirium
Compulsion	Internal pressure to engage in repetitive behavior
Concrete thinking	Mental activity without abstraction or interpretation
Confabulation	Facts are fabricated in order to disguise memory loss
Consciousness	Normal level of responsiveness to environmental events
Conversion	Dramatic physical symptoms (e.g., blindness) as a result of unconscious emotions or conflicts
Coprolalia	Impulsive expression of obscenities, as in Tourette syndrome
Countertransference	Physician's tendency to endow patients with characteristics of important people in the physician's life
Déjà vu	Feeling that one has previously experienced the same situation when one has not
Delirium	Significant clouding of consciousness
Delirium tremens	Visual hallucinations, anxiety, and autonomic hyperactivity due to alcohol withdrawal
Delusion	Fixed, false belief unresponsive to logic; not caused by ignorance or based on cultural beliefs
Dementia	Loss of cognitive abilities, especially memory
Depersonalization	Feeling of separateness from the social situation
Depression	Subjective feeling of sadness not necessarily caused by a specific loss
Derailment or loose associations	Shift of ideas from one to the other in an unrelated fashion
Derealization	Feeling that the environment is unreal or changed

Disorientation	Loss of bearings in person, place, or time
Distractibility	Problems concentrating on important stimuli
Dx	Diagnosis
DDx	Differential diagnosis
Dysarthria	Problems in articulation
Dyscalculia	Problems in ability to do simple arithmetical calculations
Dysgraphia	Problems in writing
Dysprosody	Problems using the normal rhythms of speech
Dystonia	Prolonged muscle spasms
Echolalia	Repeating another person's words over and over
Echopraxia	Repeating another person's movements over and over
Emotion	Internal psychological state
Erotomania	Delusional belief that someone is in love with you
Euphoria	Strong feelings of elation
Euthymia	Normal mood
Fetish	Inanimate object of sexual desire, such as gloves or shoes
Flat affect	Complete or almost complete lack of external emotional responsiveness
Flight of ideas	One thought follows another in quick succession, not necessarily logically
Folie à deux	Sharing of a false belief or mental state by two people; now called shared psychotic disorder
Formication	Feeling that bugs are crawling on one's skin
Free-floating anxiety	Symptoms of fear not connected to a specific cause
Fugue	Dissociative disorder with memory loss coupled with wandering away from home

Functional	Not caused by obvious organic factors
Glossolalia	Sudden ability to speak a new language (e.g., "speaking in tongues")
Gustatory	Taste
Hallucination	False sensory perception (e.g., hearing voices, smelling foul odors)
Hallucinosis	Hallucinations without delirium and associated with chronic alcoholism
Hyperphagia	Eating too much
Hypersomnia	Sleeping too much or at inappropriate times
Hypervigilance	Overconcern about external stimuli
Hypnagogic hallucination	Hallucination that occurs when falling asleep
Hypnopompic hallucination	Hallucination that occurs when waking up
Hypnosis	Modified concentration due to external suggestion, with increased focal awareness and decreased peripheral awareness
Hypochondriasis	Overconcern with physical illness
Ideas of reference	Belief that other people or the media are talking about you
Illusion	Misperception of real external stimuli (e.g., thinking a suit on a chair is a man)
Incoherence	Speech that does not make sense
Initial insomnia	Inability to fall asleep
Insight	Understanding the basis of one's own feelings and behavior
Irritable	Easily bothered and quickly angered
Jamais vu	Feeling that one has not previously experienced the same situation although one has
Kleptomania	Compulsion to steal not motivated by obvious personal gain

Labile	Rapidly changeable (opposite of stable)
Libido	Sexual interest and motivation
Loose associations	Shift of ideas from one to another in an unrelated fashion
Magical thinking	Belief that one's thoughts can change the course of events
Mood	Internal emotional feelings
Mutism (also called elective mutism)	Absence of speech despite normal physiology
Negativism	Strong resistance to suggestions of others
Neologism	Newly coined word
Neurosis	Mental disorder that affects a person's internal and external functioning but that does not involve loss of touch with reality
Orientation × 3	Patient is oriented to person, place, and time; patient knows who he is, where he is, and when it is
Obsession	Recurrent, persistent unwanted thoughts
Panic	Intense feeling of anxiety and impending doom
Paranoia	Excessive suspiciousness without adequate cause
Paraphilia	Preferential choice of unusual objects of sexual desire
Parapraxis	Slip of the tongue (i.e., "Freudian slip")
Perception	Mental interpretation of sensory stimuli
Perseveration	Continued responsiveness to a stimulus after it has been removed
Phobia	Irrational fear
Pressured speech	Rapid speech
Pseudodementia	Depression that presents with cognitive symptoms, such as memory loss and difficulty concentrating
Psychomotor agitation or retardation	Over- or under-activity due to psychological factors, often depression

Psychosis	Loss of touch with reality, characterized by hallucinations and delusions in a person with a normal level of consciousness
Reaction formation	Adopting behavior opposite to unconscious internal emotions (e.g., would-be arsonist joins a campaign to prevent forest fires)
Rationalization	Unexplainable events are explained reasonably but not convincingly to avoid intrapsychic pain (e.g., "It's a good thing they stole all my money because I would have wasted it anyway")
Reality testing	Distinguishing what is real from what is not real
Repression	Pushing unacceptable feelings out of consciousness
Restricted affect	Decreased display of emotional responsiveness
Retrograde amnesia	Lack of memory for past events, recent and remote
Rumination	Being unable to get something out of one's mind, obsessing
Rx	Treatment
Satyriasis	Insatiable need for sexual intercourse in a man
Somnambulism	Sleepwalking
Somnolence	Excessive and inappropriate sleepiness
Stereotypy	Repeated, patterned speech or actions
Stupor	Markedly decreased response to environmental stimuli
Sx	Symptom
Tactile hallucination	Sensation of being touched by or feeling something that is not there (e.g., the "phantom limb" phenomenon)
Tangentiality	Person cannot follow a train of thought to a logical conclusion, but instead gets sidetracked by unimportant issues
Terminal insomnia	Waking too early in the morning; often seen in major depressive disorder

Thought broadcasting	Feeling that one's thoughts can be heard by other people
Thought control	Feeling that one's thoughts are being manipulated by other people
Thought insertion	Feeling that other people are putting thoughts in one's head
Tic	Involuntary, sudden motor movement
Trance	Intensely focused attention, as seen in hypnosis
Transference	Patients' tendencies to endow the physician with characteristics of important people (such as parents) in the patient's life
Undoing	A defense mechanism in which past behavior is unconsciously reversed symbolically to alter something that has already occurred
Vegetative signs	Physiologic dysfunction associated with depression (e.g., insomnia or anorexia)
Verbigeration	Meaningless and repetitive talkativeness
Waxy flexibility	Like a wax figure, the patient holds any posture in which he is placed; seen in catatonic schizophrenia
Wernicke aphasia	Inability to understand speech; associated with damage to the dominant temporal lobe
Word salad	Unrelated conglomeration of words

Index

Page numbers followed by a t denote tables.